Clinics in Developmental Medicine No. 187
COMORBIDITIES IN DEVELOPMENTAL DISORDERS

T0332238

Clinics in Developmental Medicine No. 187

Comorbidities in Developmental Disorders

Edited by

MARTIN CO BAX

and

CHRISTOPHER GILLBERG

2010
Mac Keith Press

© 2010 Mac Keith Press
6 Market Road, London N7 9PW

Editor: Hilary Hart
Managing Editor: Caroline Black
Production Manager: Udoka Ohuonu
Project Manager: Mirjana Misina

First published in this edition 2010

British Library Cataloguing-in-Publication data
A catalogue record for this book is available from the British Library

Printed by Latimer Trend and Company, Plymouth
Mac Keith Press is supported by Scope

ISBN: 978-1-907655-00-5

Mac Keith Press is supported by Scope

CONTENTS

Contents

AUTHORS' APPOINTMENTS

Alan H Bittles　　Adjunct Professor and Research Leader, Centre for Comparative Genomics, Murdoch University, and Adjunct Professor of Community Genetics, School of Exercise, Biomedical and Health Sciences, Edith Cowan University, Perth, Australia

Martin CO Bax　　Honorary Reader in Child Health, Imperial College London and Honorary Consultant, Chelsea and Westminster Hospital. Dr Bax is also a Fellow of the Royal Society of Literature.

J Keith Brown　　Retired Consultant Paediatric Neurologist, Royal Hospital for Sick Children, and Fellow of University of Edinburgh, Edinburgh, UK

Sufen Chiu　　Assistant Clinical Professor, UC Davis, Sutter Center for Psychiatry, Sacramento, CA, USA

Josh Day　　Postgraduate Researcher, MIND Institute, UC Davis Medical Center, Sacramento, CA, USA

Paul Eunson　　Consultant Paediatric Neurologist, Royal Hospital for Sick Children, Edinburgh, UK

Christopher Gillberg　　Professor of Child and Adolescent Psychiatry, University of Gothenburg, Sweden and Institute of Child Health, London and Glasgow University, Glasgow, UK

Emma Glasson　　Research Assistant Professor, School of Population Health, The University of Western Australia, and School of Exercise, Biomedical and Health Sciences, Edith Cowan University, Perth, Australia

Randi Hagerman　　Professor of Pediatrics, MIND Institute UC Davis Medical Center, Sacramento, CA, USA

David Hessl　　Associate Professor, Department of Psychiatry and Behavioral Sciences and the MIND Institute, UC Davis, Sacramento, CA, USA

Brian Neville   Professor of Childhood Epilepsy, UCL Institute
                             of Child Health, Great Ormond Street Hospital,
                             London, and National Centre for Young
                             People with Epilepsy, Lingfield, Surrey, UK

Michael Orth   Consultant Neurologist, Department of
                             Neurology, Universitätskrankenhaus Ulm, Ulm,
                             Germany

Isabelle Rapin   Professor, Saul R. Korey Department of
                             Neurology, Department of Pediatrics, and
                             the Rose F. Kennedy Center for Research in
                             Mental Retardation and Human
                             Development, Albert Einstein College of
                             Medicine, Bronx, NY, USA

Mary May Robertson   Emeritus Professor of Neuropsychiatry,
                             University College London, Visiting Professor,
                             St George's Hospital Medical School, and
                             Honorary Consultant, St George's Hospital
                             Department of Mental Health Sciences,
                             University College London, London, UK

Eric Taylor   Emeritus Professor of Child and Adolescent
                             Psychiatry, Kings College London Institute of
                             Psychiatry & South London & Maudsley NHS
                             Foundation Trust, London, UK

Jeremy Turk   Professor of Developmental Psychiatry and
                             Consultant Child and Adolescent Psychiatrist,
                             Michal Rutter Centre, Maudsley Hospital,
                             Denmark Hill, London, UK

Rutger Jan Van   Professor of Psychiatry (Child & Adolescent),
der Gaag   University Medical Centre St. Radboud, and
                             Department of Psychiatry, Karakter University
                             Centre Child & Adolescent Psychiatry, Reinier,
                             Nijmegen, The Netherlands

Sameer M Zuberi   Consultant Paediatric Neurologist, Fraser of
                             Allander Neurosciences Unit, Royal Hospital
                             for Sick Children, Glasgow, UK

FOREWORD

"We think in generalities but we live in detail."
Whitehead

Working with children who have developmental disorders provides great challenges but also yields great rewards. The complex problems faced by such children and their families make it essential to take a holistic view of their care. In this book the editors Martin Bax and Christopher Gillberg have embraced these complexities. They are well placed to do so, having spent their professional lives not only looking after children who have developmental difficulties but also researching into the causes of their problems.

The editors challenge the reader to engage with the variety of disabilities associated with many disorders. There are common themes but the authors of each chapter provide insight and inspiration via the detailed analyses of the disorders they review. There are sections that discuss terminology but whilst it is important to consider, for instance, whether a disorder is comorbid or cocausal (or something else) it is also necessary to heed the advice given in the chapter on cerebral palsy: 'the child would prefer you to identify the disorder and decide what to do about it'.

It is by knowing what we are looking for that we can expect to find it. The advantage of making a diagnosis is that we can give parents and carers a prognosis based on our knowledge of particular diseases or syndromes. However, even when there is a specific diagnosis such as fragile X or Tourette syndrome the possible medical and social implications of that diagnosis are varied. It is much more difficult when a child has developmental problems of unknown cause and we may not recognise the more subtle difficulties experienced by children with attention-deficit–hyperactivity disorder or autism or epilepsy, complex groups of disorders in their own right. This book emphasises the importance of considering such variations in an individual child.

Although the determinants of behaviour are poorly understood it is increasingly recognised that behavioural phenotypes may be characteristic of particular syndromes. In the section on the channelopathies it is suggested that a single ion channel mutation may produce pathology in different tissues, thus causing comorbid neurological or behavioural disorders. This basic science research complements the empirical observations reported in other chapters, adding interest to a stimulating collection of essays by expert authors. Their descriptions of a variety of complex disorders will help the reader to identify associated problems and do something about them.

Christopher Verity
Cambridge

INTRODUCTION

Martin CO Bax and Christopher Gillberg

Towards a definition of comorbidity

In the last decade the term 'comorbidity' has gained popularity in the field of paediatric neurodisability, yet there is still no consensus about its precise definition. The definition by Feinstein, who introduced the term in his classic paper in 1970, was as follows: 'In a patient with a particular index disease, the term co-morbidity refers to any additional co-existing ailment' (note the use of the word 'ailment' rather than disease entity). This remains the definition in dictionaries and is the basis of most definitions in the published literature, particularly in the context of additional disorders that complicate the management of the index condition. However, 'comorbidity' is increasingly now used, often imprecisely and loosely, to refer to the co-occurrence of conditions more frequently than would be expected by chance, which can include instances where one condition causes the other, where they share a common cause (for example, genetic), or where they are both in fact manifestations of a single condition. Is it valid to use the term 'comorbidity' in these instances?

What is not a comorbidity?

Perhaps it would help clarify our thinking if we look at some instances which most would agree are *not* examples of comorbidity in the field of developmental medicine.

A SINGLE MORBIDITY WITH THREE SYMPTOMATOLOGIES

In a study of a whole population of five-year-olds in the Isle of Wight, a child with no reported problems was identified (Bax & Whitmore 1987). Records disclosed that the child had been seen by a cardiologist at birth because of a mild congenital thrombosis which was reviewed once a year. There was also a note that cataracts had been removed around the time of birth. The mother was impressed when the clinician queried the child's hearing, about which she was rightly concerned, the child having mild hearing loss. Clearly the clinician was correct when he made the diagnosis of rubella syndrome. The mother confirmed that she had had rubella during the pregnancy but nobody had ever mentioned it in relation to her child's problems. The morbidity here involved three different sites in the body, one cardiac, one within the orbit of the eye, and a further one relating to the functions of the 8th nerve. Both the symptomatology and the pathology varied but a single causative mechanism had been identified and a comorbidity is therefore not suggested.

A SINGLE CAUSATIVE MECHANISM WITH DIFFERENT SYMPTOMATOLOGIES?

Hypoxia produces a morbid state in the brain. The hypoxic insult affects the parts of the brain in distinct ways, white-matter damage interfering with cerebral function in a different way from damage to the grey matter. The child's symptomatology in the perinatal period is often due to one episode. But supposing a hypoxic episode occurs again two weeks late: can two episodes of hypoxia cause two different symptomatologies? If the two episodes of hypoxia cause two different symptomatologies should we regard these as comorbid states or as different symptomatologies arising from a single causative mechanisms, i.e. a single disorder?

MORE THAN ONE MORBIDITY, OR A CONDITION WITH A COMORBIDITY?

The situation is even more complex when we consider the problems that we see in the field of neurodisability. Autism can be regarded as a distinct syndromic entity. So can epilepsy. But what, then, do we make of the finding reported by Steffenburg and her colleagues (1996) of high rates of autism in a population of children identified initially because of epilepsy, whereas in a neighbouring autism clinic unknown cases of epilepsy were discovered? Both of these clinics thought that they provided a full clinical service, yet failed to identify significant pathologies: clearly the diagnoses were partly determined by which clinic a child attended. A paediatric neurologist saw the child in the epilepsy clinic, the child psychiatrist in the autism clinic. A full diagnosis would have been the first step in deciding whether to use the term 'comorbidity'. For example, if a genetic cause was identified for the autism, should the co-occurrence of epilepsy be regarded as a comorbidity or as an essential part of the basic clinical situation?

Morbidity clearly makes a person more vulnerable to a second morbidity. A viral infection will make someone more susceptible to a bacterial one and a pneumonia may develop after a 'cold', but in these circumstances it is not appropriate to use the term 'comorbid'. A child with tuberous sclerosis is quite likely to have autism or epilepsy or both. Should this be defined as one or two morbidities or a condition with a comorbidity? If learning difficulty occurs commonly in a condition, as it does in autism, most people would not label the learning disability as a comorbidity but some might: the issue is whether it shares the same aetiology as the other features of autism or whether in some way the autism predisposes the individual to learning difficulty.

COMORBIDITY OR CO-OCCURRENCE?

A child with Down syndrome with a cardiac condition is usually said to have comorbidities, whereas a child with Down syndrome and fragile X syndrome does not. The fragile X syndrome occurs at the same rate in the population with Down syndrome as it does in the typical population. Therefore, the two conditions are co-occurring at a rate that would be expected: their presence together does not relate to their aetiology. This suggests that the term 'comorbidity' could usefully be applied only when it enhances our notion of what is causing a condition rather than simply as a synonym for co-occurrence. However, our authors clearly do not all concur with this, which emphasises the lack of agreement to date and the value of the discussions in this book.

Understanding 'comorbidity': implications for aetiology, treatment and management

The contributors to this book have each grappled with the concept of comorbidity in the context of their own disciplines. Rutger Jan Van der Gaag in his chapter (pp 142–148) usefully gives examples from psychiatry to illustrate five aspects of the usage of the term comorbidity:

a) The coincidental co-occurrence of two distinct conditions (e.g. pneumonia requiring treatment in a patient in hospital for a psychosis);

b) two different aspects of one condition that might require attention in their own right (e.g. anxiety and sleep problems in a depression);

c) the frequent co-occurrence of two conditions, with a possible unknown relationship between them, without speculating on the nature of that relationship;

d) a causal relationship;

e) a time-development-track interaction.

Brown and Eunson in their chapter on cerebral palsy (pp 20–39) provide a thorough review of all the 'associated conditions' that may accompany the index condition cerebral palsy. Their definition of a comorbidity is that it is any condition which is associated with the index condition, and which can appear as an entity in its own right. As they comment, however, the difficulty in child neurology is that many of the major conditions, such as hearing difficulty, epilepsy, cerebral palsy, attention deficit disorder, hyperkinetic syndrome and autism, are not disease entities but syndromes, all arising from brain dysfunction. They go on to propose that there is a useful distinction to be made between three kinds of association: comorbid disorders, co-causal disorders, and complications of the index condition. Thus whereas some comorbid conditions are neither caused by nor complications of the cerebral palsy, other conditions have the same aetiology (brain dysfunction); this is an example of a *co-causal* association. They distinguish other conditions such as constipation as *complications* of the cerebral palsy.

Zuberi's account of co-morbidities in the context of channelopathies (pp 116–124) is also helpful in establishing a possible explanation for some comorbidities. He points out that somewhat similar presentations in these channelopathies might make one wonder if there is a single morbid cause but in fact a range of genes is causing the symptomatologies. Conversely, Zuberi presents examples of instances where a single ion channel mutation producing pathology in different tissues could be the explanation for co-morbid neurological or behavioural disorders in an individual. These findings are clearly interesting in relation to the issue of comorbidity but they are also important in terms of the development of new treatments.

Bittles' (pp 125–141) discussion of a new symptomatology emerging 'with age' poses another set of problems: do we accept a symptomatology developing later in life as part of the original diagnostic concept or is it perhaps a comorbidity? The issue arises with Down syndrome: most people would accept that the early onset of dementia is caused by the same aetiological factors as the original learning difficulty. Bittles makes us put 'time' into our equation. One might question whether what he describes in older children is part of the original morbidity, is a comorbidity, or is a completely different phenomenon co-occurring with the index condition.

Can the presence of comorbidities that occur more often than would be expected by chance tell us something about the aetiology of a condition? Clinicians have for years been constantly surprised that the classic symptoms of one condition can be associated with those of another condition thought to be distinct and different. These are not part of the same disorder but they co-occur. Orth and Robertson in their chapter (pp 40–59) refer to a study in which the classic signs of Tourette syndrome – the tic-like behaviours – occurred alone in only about 10% of those who had been diagnosed with this syndrome. In the other individuals there was at least one comorbidity. They note that it is not yet clear whether Tourette syndrome and its common co-occurring disorders – such as attention-deficit–hyperactivity disorder and obsessive-compulsive disorder – are true co-morbidities, or whether they have a common genetic and/or environmental cause. As these disorders are all common their combination could be a chance co-occurrence. However, their co-occurrence is so frequent that they probably share aetiologically relevant factors. What do we mean if we use 'comorbidity' in these circumstances? In future would we use the label 'Tourette syndrome' to describe a set of symptoms as we do now or should we simply describe the presenting behaviour?

When we describe a condition we hope that this will lead us to identify a cause, whether genetic, traumatic, infective, degenerative or neoplastic. We diagnose a 'disease' when we know the cause of the condition and its course, symptomatology and consequences. A 'syndrome' is a cluster of symptoms and signs which often occur together: for example, an association between individuals who have tics and those who have coprolalia seems rational because these behaviours have often been noted together and they are both impulsive and uncontrollable behaviours. It may be, however, that the 'tic' behaviour alone, with its various possible causes, should be regarded in isolation, and the notion of a disease entity 'Tourette syndrome' should be abandoned.

Conclusion

The extensive range of manifestations seen in all the conditions discussed in this book would be depressing reading for many parents, who are often not aware of the implications of the original diagnosis. When we counsel parents on the future of their child our predictions will be better in individual patients when we know of genetic factors or signs which will allow us to recognize how particular children will develop. For the moment, perhaps the identification of comorbidities and other co-occurring events increases our knowledge but perhaps also increases our perplexities in knowing what to do in a situation and how best to help parents. We hope that this book will help the clinician discuss with parents what is happening to their children and explain the rationale of any treatment which is being devised.

It became clear to us as we collated the chapters for this book that we were not going to establish a clear agreed definition of what a comorbidity is. What we present is a stimulating set of essays on topics that the authors know well and where they, within the framework they had set themselves, wrestled with how they use the term 'comorbid'.

Indeed, what has become manifest is that many people with great experience in the field of neurodisability have slightly different concepts of the term. We have no doubt that others in the field will find these discussions of great interest.

REFERENCES

Bax M, Whitmore K (1987) The medical examination of children on entry to school. The results and use of neurodevelopmental assessment. *Dev Med Child Neurol*, **29**, 40–55.
Feinstein A (1970) The pre-therapeutic classification of co-morbidity in chronic disease. *J Chron Dis*, **23**, 455–468.
Steffenburg S, Gillberg C, Steffenburg U. Psychiatric disorders in children and adolescents with mental retardation and active epilepsy. *Arch Neurol* 1996, **53**, 904–912.

This book was inspired by a study group of international experts drawn together by the Castang Foundation to discuss the concept of comorbidity and how it can contribute to the understanding and management of developmental disorders. Their deliberations are augmented by those of some additional contributors chosen to broaden the breadth of the book.

1
INTELLECTUAL DISABILITIES AND THEIR COMORBIDITIES

Jeremy Turk

Intellectual disability refers to early-onset and long-term generalised impairments in intellectual functioning. These impairments are of a global nature (American Association on Mental Retardation 2002). They may comprise slowness in development with a significantly lower than average final level of intellectual functioning (retardation) or distortions of the developmental process – so-called 'qualitative impairments'. Often they comprise both together. These intellectual disabilities are associated with functional impairments in social, adaptive and other important life skills (Hatton 1998). They render the individual reliant on others, to a degree, in order to experience a reasonable quality of life free from avoidable secondary restrictions and exploitation. Standard diagnostic criteria of the *International Classification of Diseases* (ICD) of the World Health Organization (WHO 1992) and the *Diagnostic and Statistical Manual* (DSM) of the American Psychiatric Association (American Psychiatric Association 1994) stipulate the need for intellectual functioning as measured by standardised psychometric tests to be at least two standard deviations below the mean. Thus, for the usual model of a normal Gaussian distribution of intelligence within the general population, with a mean of 100 intellectual quotient (IQ) points and a standard deviation of 15 IQ points, individuals must score no greater than 70 in order to qualify for a label of ICD or DSM 'Mental Retardation', synonymous with the term 'intellectual disability' as used in this book. Hence, at any time, 2–3% of the population will have an IQ consistent with having intellectual disability. Moderate-to-profound intellectual disability (IQ less than 50) occurs in 3–4 per 1000 individuals (Abramowicz & Richardson 1975). However, only a proportion of those with intellectual disability will experience the functional impairments and associated social disabilities and disadvantages necessary to warrant the *clinical* label and to require professional support.

Terminology

Preference for the label 'intellectual disability' is more than cosmetic. First, it is gaining ever increasing international popularity as a term for this particular client group's difficulties and special needs. Indeed, the two leading European academic publications in this field, the *Journal of Intellectual Disability Research* and the *Journal of Applied Research in Intellectual Disabilities*, have for a time favoured this terminology. Second, the phrase avoids derogatory connotations associated with earlier labels, not only archaic ones such as idiot, imbecile and feeble-minded but more recent abbreviations and corruptions, for example subnormal, retardate, cretin and spastic. Third, it avoids confusions between English usage of the term 'learning disability' (to mean generalised intellectual disability) and North American usage (to mean specific learning difficulties or specific developmental delays such as dyslexia, dyscalculia and dysgraphia). Fourth, audits and surveys of client group preferences confirm almost unanimous dislike for terms such as mental retardation, mental impairment and mental handicap. Service users argue that the term 'mental' leads too readily to confusion with serious psychiatric disorders such as schizophrenia and manic-depressive psychosis. Most individuals with intellectual disability do not suffer with such disorders although rates are certainly higher than in the general population for a number of biological, psychological and social reasons (Rutter et al. 1970, Emerson 2003, Ford et al. 2003). Furthermore, use of the term 'disability' shifts focus away from the underlying impairment which may be structural (such as brain damage through hypoxia, physical trauma or neurodevelopmental defect) or psychological (such as problem solving, executive function or information-processing limitations) but which is usually (but not always) immutable. It is the functional consequences of impairments which can be worked on in order to minimise disability and participation restriction and maximise potential.

Intellectual disability, in health terminology, can be mild (equivalent to a rough IQ estimate of 50–70), moderate (rough IQ estimate of 35–50), severe (rough IQ estimate of 20–35) or profound (rough IQ estimate of less than 20 IQ points). There is no particular preference for certain socio-economic, cultural or racial backgrounds.

Unhelpfully but importantly, educational terminology, at least in the United Kingdom, is based on a different classification termed 'learning difficulties'. In this scenario, moderate learning difficulties denotes a rough IQ estimate of 50–70, while severe learning difficulties denotes a rough IQ estimate of less than 50. The potential confusions are obvious, for example when a clinician describes mild intellectual disability only for this to be mistaken for low average intellectual functioning by educationalists. See Turk (1996), Turk et al. (2007) and Bernard et al. (2009) for further discussions of terminology and its implications.

Features associated with intellectual disability

Having intellectual disability is associated with a range of increased complications and needs. These include physical, psychiatric, social, linguistic, financial, economic, political and not least neurodevelopmental aspects (Turk 1997).

Physical comorbidities are more common in people with intellectual disability than in the general population. They may comprise characteristic appearances such as the facies in Down syndrome (Marder & Dennis 2001), the port wine facial stain indicative of intracranial cavernous haemangiomata in Sturge–Weber syndrome (Comi 2003), the elfin-like facial appearance in Williams syndrome (Tarjan et al. 2003), the jerky ataxic gait and open mouth in Angelman syndrome (Clayton-Smith & Laan 2003) and the longish, largish head with large chin, high-arched palate and simple protruding ears with postpubertal macroorchidism, widespread ligamentous laxity and joint hypermobility frequently witnessed in fragile X syndrome (Hagerman 1996).

Sensory problems are also more frequent amongst people with intellectual disability than those of average intelligence, in particular visual and auditory difficulties (Turk &

Patton 2000). They are even more common and pronounced in some specific genetic syndromes which cause intellectual disability. Examples include the raised rate of conductive and sensorineural hearing loss, refractory visual errors and squint in Down syndrome, and the hyperacusis (auditory sensitivity) characteristic of Williams syndrome (van Borsel et al. 1997, Metcalfe 1999). Associated motor function impairments are common in conditions where intellectual disability co-occurs with cerebellar, brainstem and spinal cord anomalies. Examples include hydrocephalus, spina bifida, Joubert syndrome (congenital cerebellar vermis hypoplasia) (Merritt 2003) and Arnold–Chiari malformation (persistence of embryological cerebellar tonsils herniating through the foramen magnum) (Arnett 2003).

Social and linguistic comorbidities are common, as witnessed by the relationship between intellectual disability and autistic spectrum disorder. The rates of autism spectrum disorders in children with intellectual disability are substantially raised (Nordin & Gillberg 1996). Up to 50% of individuals with moderate to profound intellectual disability have an autistic spectrum disorder (Wing & Gould 1979) and the degree of intellectual disability is related to the likelihood of having an autistic spectrum disorder and severity of autistic features. Conversely, 70% of children on the autistic spectrum have a non-verbal IQ below 70 and 50% of children on the autistic spectrum have a non-verbal IQ below 50 while only about 5% of children on the autistic spectrum have an IQ above 100 (high functioning autism).

The general rate of *psychiatric disorder* in people with intellectual disability is raised, both in childhood (Rutter et al. 1970, Emerson 2003) and in adults. Epilepsy has a substantially greater prevalence in populations with intellectual disability (Jansen et al. 2004). Furthermore, the combination of epilepsy and intellectual disability produces substantially higher rates of psychopathology (Steffenburg et al. 1996, Espie et al. 2003). Cerebral palsy, too, is more common in people with intellectual disability (Arvio & Sillanpaa 2003). Again, having intellectual disability and cerebral palsy combined produces further elevated rates of psychiatric disorder as does the combination of having autism and epilepsy (Turk et al. 2009).

The key to a comprehensive understanding of comorbidities in the field of intellectual disability is an appreciation that intelligence defines only one of many dimensions of mental life and mental development. These dimensions can be viewed as modular – that is to say that although impairments in one frequently coincide with impairments in others, this is not always the case. Extreme examples include the catastrophic social and language impairments with associated personality difficulties, obsessions and rigidities coexisting with at least average intellectual ability in individuals with high-functioning autism and Asperger syndrome (Koning & Magill-Evans 2001, Soderstrom et al. 2002), and the shyness, social anxiety, attentional deficits, numeracy difficulties, visuospatial problems and executive function deficits witnessed in fragile X premutation carriers, even those with good general intellectual abilities (Aziz et al. 2003).

Thus intellectual disability is associated with multiple comorbidities spanning multiple domains of both physical and mental life and functioning. These comorbidities all have multiple possible causes and multiple inter-relationships and interactions with other developmental dimensions.

Reasons for psychiatric and psychological comorbidities

There is a range of reasons why psychological difficulties may be associated with intellectual disability. First, the co-occurring emotional or behavioural state, or 'challenging behaviour', may be consistent with the individual's general developmental level of abilities. For example, it would be unreasonable to expect a 10 year old with an IQ of approximately 50 to have social, linguistic and attentional skills that differ significantly from those of an average 5 year old. The fact that these attributes exist in an individual of substantially greater stature and strength may well in itself produce social if not clinical issues, and all the more so as the individual enters adolescence and puberty. However, understanding of the developmental 'normality' of such behavioural traits can help considerably in the creation of rational and realistic intervention and support strategies.

Secondly, the individual's presenting psychiatric, psychological and behavioural challenges may reflect emotional reactions to experiences common to us all, such as bereavement (Hollins & Esterhuyzen 1997), other losses, anticipatory anxieties, reactions to unexpected or overwhelming change in surroundings or routine, abuse and neglect (Turk & Brown 1993), being misunderstood by others, and other life events and daily hassles (Ghaziuddin 1988). In such situations care must be taken not to fall into the trap of diagnostic overshadowing, whereby all behavioural and other challenges are attributed to the individual having intellectual disability, with the therapeutic fatalism and nihilism inherent in such a perspective.

Thirdly, it is important to remember that an individual with generalised intellectual disability is still prone (indeed, more so than the general population) to specific developmental delays. These may be attentional, social, linguistic, obsessive-compulsive, sensory and motor. They are often multiple. At their most extreme, they can qualify the individual for further diagnoses such as attention-deficit–hyperactivity disorder (ADHD) (Ishii et al. 2003), autism spectrum disorder (Howlin 2000) or dyspraxia. Diagnosis of such associated specific developmental delays in the presence of generalised intellectual disability is certainly more complicated than is usually the case. However, it is all the more important given the potential for misunderstandings and misattributions regarding causality (for example, mistaking a neurodevelopmental delay for inept parenting, abuse or neglect, or personal malice), and the fact that often the difficulties are amenable to the same battery of evidence-based medical, psychological, educational and social interventions as apply to those without generalised intellectual disability.

Aetiologically, the common neuropsychiatric and neurodevelopmental disorders frequently witnessed in association with intellectual disability (i.e. ADHD and autism spectrum disorders) seem to be part of a common genetic predisposition whereby whatever the genetic basis of the intellectual disability, there are substantially increased rates of ADHD and autistic spectrum disorders, with the curious exceptions of Down syndrome and Prader–Willi syndrome, in particular the *unipaternal disomy* form (Åkefeldt & Gillberg 1999, Veltman et al. 2004). However, it is important to note that the rates of ADHD and autism spectrum disorder in individuals with trisomy 21 Down syndrome and Prader–Willi syndrome are substantially greater than in the general population. Nevertheless, they are lower than expected given the levels of intellectual functioning of Down syndrome and Prader–Willi syndrome individuals (Green et al. 1989, Rasmussen et al. 2001).

Finally, such neurobehavioural disabilities and disorders may be specific to particular conditions, when they form part of the so-called *behavioural phenotype* (O'Brien 2002). A well-recognised example is the compulsive extreme self-injury in individuals with Lesch–Nyhan syndrome, an X-linked genetic disorder resulting in absence of the enzyme 5-hypoxanthine guanine phosphoribosyl transferase (5HGPRT) which is critical in the metabolism of urate (Robey et al. 2003). Another well-researched association is the voracious overeating (hyperphagia) and obesity in association with unpredictable tantrumming and skin picking found in individuals with Prader–Willi syndrome, due to anomalies on the long arm of chromosome 15 (Descheemaeker et al. 2002). These behaviours replace early floppiness, feeble feeding and failure to thrive, emphasising the importance of developmental trajectories in understanding the nature of neurodevelopmental comorbidities and behavioural phenotypes and their relationships to intellectual disability. A third well-documented illustration is the relentless cognitive deterioration with development of autistic tendencies, spinal curvature (scoliosis), respiratory compromise, overbreathing and midline 'hand wringing' stereotypies following an initial phase of apparently normal development in individuals with Rett syndrome (Colvin et al. 2003). This is associated with a micro-deletion towards the tip of the X chromosome's long arm, involving the MecP2 gene (Christodoulou & Weaving 2003). The *hemizygous* state (XY) is incompatible with life, such conceptions usually resulting in early miscarriage. The *heterozygous* state (XX), with one of the two X chromosomes bearing the Rett syndrome genetic anomaly, is usually compatible with life yet results in this devastating neurodevelopmental disability.

Down syndrome: an illustration of a specific aetiological cause of intellectual disability associated with a characteristic profile of comorbidities

Down syndrome is the most common cause of intellectual disability, occurring in approximately one in 650 livebirths (Selikowitz 1997). The vast majority of individuals have the trisomy 21 non-inherited variant, the main risk factor being increased maternal age. A small minority have a translocation variant which is inherited, emphasising the importance of chromosomal analysis of all newborn infants with Down syndrome, even when the clinical features and diagnosis are obvious, in order that familial genetic counselling can be undertaken where appropriate (Jyothy et al. 2002). The average level of intellectual functioning of people with Down syndrome is in the moderate-to-severe intellectual disability range (Carr 1988). However, the distribution remains statistically normal with 'outliers' at either end. The normal multifactorial (polygenic plus multiple environmental influences) distribution of intelligence has been 'shifted down' by the influence of a third chromosome 21. Thus, even in the population of people with Down syndrome, there are those who are 'brighter', functioning within the low average intelligence range, yet equally those with particularly special needs often compromising profound and multiple disabilities that lie cognitively at the other end of the intelligence distribution.

A further complication in Down syndrome is the occasional presence of mosaicism. In this situation, a proportion of the cells in the body and brain of an individual with Down syndrome carry the normal complement of 46 chromosomes. In such instances the degree of physical and psychological affectedness is determined by the proportion of cells carrying the trisomy 21 anomaly. Greater proportions of such cells are associated with more severe levels of intellectual disability and more pronounced physical features.

There is little evidence for a particularly uneven cognitive profile in those with Down syndrome. However, adaptive behaviours and social skills, at least early on in development, may be relatively precocious, to the extent of belying the severity of intellectual disability (Dykens et al. 2002). Langdon Down's early anecdotal descriptions of a characteristic personality profile of friendliness, sociability, affection and love of music have to an extent been confirmed by more recent scientific studies, suggesting that there is indeed a characteristic personality and temperamental profile in people with Down syndrome (Gibbs & Thorpe 1983) even though the applicability of well-established personality and temperament scales to populations with intellectual disability may be in doubt (Gibbs et al. 1987).

The relatively low rates of autistic spectrum disorders and attention-deficit disorders in children with Down syndrome have already been alluded to. However, this can mean that when autistic disorders do coexist with Down syndrome, as they may in 10% of instances (as opposed to the much higher rate expected in a group with an average IQ in the moderate-to-profound intellectual disability range), then this important association is missed clinically (Kent et al. 1999).

A further concerning neurodevelopmental twist has been the confirmation of raised rates of clinical depression in adolescents and young adults with Down syndrome, even when level of intellectual functioning, chronological age, social environment, life events and daily hassles have been controlled for (Collacott et al. 1998). This, along with the now well-recognised association between Down syndrome and early-onset Alzheimer presenile dementia (Dodd et al. 2005), means that apparent cognitive decline, social and behavioural withdrawal, and diminishing interest in previously enjoyed activities and pastimes require particularly careful evaluation and appropriate supports.

Frequent clinical common final pathways

The example of Down syndrome illustrates the truism that any one cause of intellectual disability may be associated with a large number of phenomenological end-states – and any number of these may coexist in one individual. The opposite is also true, i.e. that any one phenomenological end-state may be associated with a large number of causes. Illustrative examples of this include ADHD, autistic spectrum disorders and self-injurious tendencies.

Traditionally, there have been considered to be two major determinants of the likelihood and severity of psychological and psychiatric disorders in individuals with intellectual disability, namely degree of intellectual impairment and the quality of the individual's social environment and upbringing (Rutter et al. 1970). These two variables are certainly critical in determining likelihood and severity of emotional and behavioural disturbance. However, to them we must now add aetiology of intellectual disability as a further cause, not just genetic but infective (e.g. congenital rubella (Carvill & Marston 2002)), toxic (e.g. fetal alcohol syndrome (Aronson et al. 1997, Lee et al. 2004)), iatrogenic (e.g. congenital anticonvulsant exposure syndromes (Dean et al. 2002)) and possibly psychosocial as in the predicament of Romanian orphans starved of emotional and social stimulation at critical times in development (Chugani et al. 2001). Furthermore, there is a need to consider interactions, gene–gene (epistasis), gene–environment and even environment–environment, where one variable may ameliorate potentially adverse other variables (resilience factors) or may aggravate them (complicating or exacerbating factors).

Self-injury

There is no doubt that the likelihood and severity of self-injury in people with intellectual disability is largely determined by psychological and social issues and contingencies (Oliver 1995). However, it is equally true that the likelihood and severity of self-injurious tendencies increase as level of intellectual disability becomes more severe (McClintock et al. 2003). Additionally, self-injury may be the presenting feature in a number of specific genetically determined intellectual disability syndromes. In these instances, the nature or content of the self-injury is remarkably aetiology specific. Lesch–Nyhan syndrome is consistently associated with extreme compulsive and distressing gnawing and biting of knuckles to the extent of skin and underlying tendon erosion (Hall et al. 2001). Restraint is often welcomed by sufferers despite many practitioners' ethical aversion to its use. Examples of ingenious self-restraint and self-control strategies developed by sufferers to modulate their self-destructive compulsions have been reported (Oliver et al. 2003). In Cornelia de Lange syndrome, hyperactive tendencies and moderate-to-severe intellectual disability is associated with lip biting (Berney et al. 1999). In fragile X syndrome the self-injury usually takes the form of biting at the base of the thumb over the 'anatomical snuff-box' in response to anxiety or excitement (Symons et al. 2003). Prader–Willi syndrome predisposes to self-destructive overeating which commonly exacerbates and complicates the raised incidence of diabetes mellitus, as well as compulsive picking at already delicate and fragile skin (Descheemaeker et al. 2002). Smith–Magenis syndrome (Smith et al. 1998), attributable to a microdeletion on the short arm of chromosome 17, leads not only to intellectual disability but also to catastrophic sleep disturbance, gross inattentiveness and overactivity, autistic tendencies and extreme self-injury, usually in the forms of pulling out finger and toenails (onychotillomania) and inserting objects compulsively and repetitively into bodily orifices (polyembolokoilomania).

Reasons for this high specificity of type of self-injury in relation to genetic aetiology remain obscure and poorly understood. However, it seems clear that while likelihood, situationality and severity of self-injury are influenced substantially by psychosocial and in particular behavioural factors, the nature (and probably likelihood and severity) of self-injury is influenced considerably by neurodevelopmental aetiology.

The need for a conceptual shift

Historically there has been a trend for all people with intellectual disability to be considered as one homogeneous grouping, as suggested by early publications exploring the emotional and behavioural disturbances experienced by individuals with intellectual disability (e.g. Phillips & Williams 1975, Groden et al. 1982, Koller et al. 1983). We are now in a position to commence a move from all-or-nothing, discrete, categorical, phenomenologically based classifications, such as 'mental retardation', towards multidimensional, aetiologically driven classifications of developmental disabilities which allow pinpointing of each individual in multidimensional space in terms of not just intellectual but also social, linguistic, attentional, sensory and motor functioning. To an extent, this movement has already commenced in terms of the multiaxial classificatory model's acknowledgement of the importance of not just psychiatric diagnosis but also coexisting specific developmental delays, level of general intellectual functioning, associated medical conditions, important psychosocial circumstances and experiences, and degree of functional impairment. However, a conceptual step further is required in order to acknowledge that aetiology of the individual's intellectual disability is important in determining not only severity of intellectual impairment but also profile of cognitive strengths and needs, associated developmental abilities and disabilities, developmental trajectories, and thus psychosocial associations. There is evidence that 'genes drive behaviour' (Scarr & McCartney 1983), that there are substantial genetic influences on temperament, personality and other psychological traits (Reif & Lesch 2003), and that these influences increase rather than decrease with age and experience (Plomin 1988).

Example of multidimensional aetiologically driven developmental and psychological profiles: fragile X syndrome

Fragile X syndrome is the most common identifiable cause of inherited intellectual disability, occurring in approximately 1 in 4000 livebirths (Hagerman & Cronister 1996). It has equal prevalence rates in all races and cultures worldwide. It is caused by an abnormal DNA expansion just above the tip of the X chromosome's long arm. This results in impaired production of the fragile X mental retardation 1 protein (FMRP) which is known to contain chemical sequences consistent with the roles of nucleus–cytoplasm transfer of messenger RNA and messenger RNA–ribosomal binding. It thus has important 'housekeeping' roles in terms of facilitating functioning of other protein-producing genes, presumably including at least some critical to neurodevelopment. There are a number of associated physical features (see Hagerman 1996, Turk & Patton 2000) but none of these is pathognomonic of the condition, all occur in other genetic disorders and indeed are seen in many members of the general population. However, a substantial number of research publications confirm the existence of a characteristic cognitive, psychological and behavioural phenotype with important developmental trajectories and clinical implications (Cornish et al. 2004).

Intellectual functioning is usually in the mild-to-moderate intellectual disability range. There is an uneven cognitive profile whereby relative linguistic strengths belie numeracy and visuospatial difficulties, even in those with average-range general intellectual abilities. Discrepancy between cognitive skills of those with fragile X syndrome and non-intellectually disabled peers increases as individuals approach adolescence (Fisch et al. 1996). This is attributable to specific difficulties with sequential (as opposed to simultaneous) information processing. Executive function difficulties have been noted in female carriers and male premutation carriers (Loesch et al. 2003). These manifest as concentration and attentional problems, difficulties in shifting from one topic to another, impaired problem-solving abilities, poor organisational skills and trouble with planning abilities.

Speech and language (Cornish et al. 2004, Taylor 2004) often have a humorous quality with up and down (litanic) swings of pitch, perseverations and repetitiveness, delayed echolalia and cluttering, a mixture of rapid and dysrhythmic speech components.

As many as 28% of young boys with fragile X syndrome have ICD-10 childhood autism. A larger proportion has a characteristic profile of multiple social and language autistic impairments in the presence of a friendly and sociable, albeit shy and socially avoidant personality (Turk & Graham 1997). There is an aversion to eye contact as exhibited in exaggerated avoidance postures during greeting (Garrett et al. 2004), self-injury in the form of hand biting in response to anxiety and excitement (Symons et al. 2003), delays in the development of imitative and symbolic play (Rogers et al. 2003) and a tendency toward stereotyped and repetitive behaviours, including hand flapping and insistence on routine (Turk & Graham 1997). These usually exist in the presence of good understanding of facial expression and theory of mind development consistent with general level of intellectual ability (Turk & Cornish 1998). Recent research findings suggest that rates of diagnosable autistic spectrum disorder increase substantially with age, although the exact reasons for this finding remain unresolved (Turk et al. 2003).

Attentional deficits are common, as are poor concentration, restlessness, fidgetiness, impulsiveness, distractibility and overactivity. Gross motor activity is not necessarily greater than expected for age and developmental abilities, but the other described features usually persist and often require medical and psychological intervention (Turk 1998).

Pilot work on young women with fragile X full mutations and premutations suggests that they too can show a wide range of affectedness, with autism spectrum disorders and ADHD being common even in the presence of reasonable intellectual functioning. Similarly, boys and men with fragile X premutations can experience important developmental difficulties socially, linguistically and attentionally (Aziz et al. 2003, Cornish et al. 2004). Also, the rate of diagnosable DSM-IV autistic disorder has been found to double in young adult men compared with preadolescent and early adolescent boys (Turk et al. 2003).

Conspicuousness by absence

It is of equal importance to note that specific aetiologies of intellectual disability need not predispose to developmental neuropsychiatric disturbances For example, Down syndrome is associated with surprisingly low rates of autistic spectrum and attention-deficit disorders given the general distribution of intelligence amongst individuals with the condition (Dykens et al. 2002). Individuals with Prader–Willi syndrome have similar if not lower rates of autistic spectrum and attention-deficit disorders, although they do have other psychological difficulties (Descheemaeker et al. 2002). FraX-E, a rare form of fragile X syndrome with its own discrete DNA expansion abnormality towards the X chromosome's tip, was initially thought to have a behavioural phenotype manifesting as a mild version of that seen in FraX-A, the 'common' form of fragile X syndrome (Barnicoat et al. 1997, Freeman & Turk, 2007). However, more recent studies suggest that individuals with FraX-E can have extremely variable levels of intellectual functioning ranging from average to severe/profound intellectual disability, and that the presence of autistic spectrum disorder can be equally variable, calling into question whether this particular condition has a behavioural phenotype at all (May et al. 2003).

15

Conclusion

In conclusion, it is evident that the presence of comorbid physical, psychiatric, psychological and behavioural disorders in individuals with intellectual disability is common, and more frequently witnessed than in those of more average intellectual ability. The occurrence of neurodevelopmental disorders (such as autism and ADHD) as comorbidities may even be the rule rather than the exception, particularly for those with moderate-to-profound intellectual disability. These comorbidities cover the entire biopsychosocial spectrum and can be attributed to the same causative agents as the intellectual impairments that they accompany. One practical consequence of this is that the educational needs of an individual with, say, severe intellectual disability and autism can only be met in a school environment expert in meeting the needs of students with both sets of neurodevelopmental challenges, not one or the other. In short, both intellectual disabilities and the comorbidities discussed in this chapter are common final clinical pathways with multiple possible causes and multiple possible combinations and permutations. These multiple causes and their combinations in any one individual contribute significantly to the nature of the developmental difficulties experienced and hence have substantial implications for intervention, as witnessed by publications focusing on the educational needs of students with particular genetic conditions (e.g. Lorenz 1998, Waters 1999, Dew-Hughes 2003). These multiple interactions of the biological, psychological and social are common and important diagnostically, therapeutically and amelioratively.

REFERENCES

Abramowicz HK, Richardson SA (1975) Epidemiology of severe mental retardation in children: community studies. *Am J Mental Retard* **80**, 18–39.

Åkefeldt A, Gillberg C (1999) Behavior and personality characteristics of children and young adults with Prader-Willi syndrome: a controlled study. *J Am Coll Child Adolesc Psychiatr* **38**, 761–769.

American Association on Mental Retardation (2002) *Mental Retardation: Definition, Classification and Systems of Supports*. Washington, DC: American Association on Mental Retardation.

American Psychiatric Association (1994) *Diagnostic and Statistical Manual of Mental Disorders*, 4th edn. Washington, DC: American Psychiatric Association.

Arnett B (2003) Arnold–Chiari malformation. *Arch Neurol* **60**, 898–900.

Aronson M, Hagberg B, Gillberg C (1997) Attention deficits and autistic spectrum problems in children exposed to alcohol during gestation: a follow-up study. *Dev Med Child Neurol* 39, 583–587.

Arvio M, Sillanpaa M (2003) Prevalence, aetiology and comorbidity of severe and profound intellectual disability in Finland. *J Intellect Disabil Res* 47, 108–112.

Aziz M, Stathopulu E, Callias M, et al. (2003) Clinical features of boys with fragile X premutations and intermediate alleles. *Am J Med Genet B: Neuropsychiatr Genet* 121B, 119–127.

Barnicoat AJ, Wang Q, Turk J, et al. (1997) Clinical, cytogenetic, and molecular analysis of three families with FRAXE. *J Med Genet* **34**, 13–17.

Bernard S, Turk J (2009) *Developing Mental Health Services for Children & Adolescents with Learning Disabilities; a Toolkit for Clinicians*. London: Royal College of Psychiatrists.

Berney TP, Ireland M, Burn J. (1999) Behavioural phenotype of Cornelia de Lange syndrome. *Arch Dis Child* **81**, 333–336.

Carr J (1988) Six weeks to twenty-one years old: a longitudinal study of children with Down's syndrome and their families. *J Child Psychol Psychiatr* **29**, 407–432.

Carvill S, Marston G (2002) People with intellectual disability, sensory impairments and behaviour disorder: a case series. *J Intellect Disabil Res* 46, 264–272.

Christodoulou J, Weaving LS (2003) MECP2 and beyond: phenotype-genotype correlations in Rett syndrome. *J Child Neurol* **18**, 669–674.

Chugani HT, Behen ME, Muzik O, et al. (2001) Local brain functional activity following early deprivation: a study of postinstitutionalized Romanian orphans. *Neuroimage* **14**, 1290–1301.

Clayton-Smith J, Laan L (2003) Angelman syndrome: a review of the clinical and genetic aspects. *J Med Genet* **40**, 87–95.

Collacott RA, Cooper SA, Branford D, Mcgrother C (1998) Behaviour phenotype for Down's syndrome. *Br J Psychiatr* **172**, 85–89.

Colvin L, Fyfe S, Leonard S, et al. (2003) Describing the phenotype of Rett syndrome using a population database. *Arch Dis Child* **88**, 38–43.

Comi AM (2003) Pathophysiology of Sturge–Weber syndrome. *J Child Neurol* **18**, 509–16,

Cornish K, Sudhalter V, Turk J (2004) Attention and language in fragile X. *Mental Retard Dev Disabil Res Rev* 10, 11–16.

Dean JC, Hailey H, Moore S, et al. (2002) Long term health and neurodevelopment in children exposed to antiepileptic drugs before birth. *J Med Genet* **39**, 251–259.

Descheemaeker MJ, Vogels A, Govers V, et al. (2002) Prader–Willi syndrome: new insights in the behavioural and psychiatric spectrum. *J Intellect Disabil Res* **46**, 41–50.

Dew-Hughes D (2003) *Educating Children with Fragile X Syndrome*. London: Routledge Falmer.

Dodd k, Turk V, Christmas M (2005) *Down's Syndrome And Dementia Resource Pack For Carers And Support Staff*. Kidderminster: BILD Publications.

Dykens EM, Shah B, Sagun J, Beck T, King BH (2002) Maladaptive behaviour in children and adolescents with Down's syndrome. *J Intellect Disabil Res* **46**, 484–492.

Emerson E (2003) Prevalence of psychiatric disorders in children and adolescents with and without intellectual disability. *J Intellect Disabil Res* **47**, 51–58.

Espie CA, Watkins J, Curtice L, et al. (2003) Psychopathology in people with epilepsy and intellectual disability; an investigation of potential explanatory variables. *J Neurol Neurosurg Psychiatr* **74**, 1485–1492.

Fisch GS, Simensen R, Tarleton J (1996) Longitudinal study of cognitive abilities and adaptive behaviour levels in fragile X males: a prospective multicenter analysis. *Am J Med Genet* **64**, 356–361.

Ford T, Goodman R, Meltzer H (2003) The British Child and Adolescent Mental Health Survey 1999: the prevalence of DSM-IV disorders. *J Am Acad Child Adolesc Psychiatr* **42**, 1203–1211.

Freeman L, Turk J (2007) FraX-E: underdiagnosed, undertreated, under-researched & misunderstood? *Advances in Mental Health in Learning Disabilities* **1**, 40–51.

Garrett AS, Menon V, MacKenzie K, Reiss AL (2004) Here's looking at you kid: neural systems underlying face and gaze processing in fragile X syndrome. *Arch Gen Psychiatr* **61**, 281–288.

Ghaziuddin M (1988) Behavioural disorder in the mentally handicapped. The role of life events. *Br J Psychiatr* **152**, 683–686.

Gibbs MV, Thorpe JG (1983) Personality stereotype of noninstitutionalised Down syndrome children. *Am J Mental Defic* **87**, 601–605.

Gibbs MV, Reeves D, Cunningham CC (1987) The application of temperament questionnaires to a British sample: issues of reliability and validity. *J Child Psychol Psychiatr* **28**, 61–77.

Graham PJ, Turk J, Verhulst F (1999) *Child Psychiatry: A Developmental Approach*, 3rd edn. Oxford: Oxford University Press.

Green JM, Dennis J, Bennets LA (1989) Attention disorder in a group of young Down's syndrome children. *J Mental Defic Res* **33**, 105–122.

Groden G, Domingue D, Pueschel SM, Deignan L (1982) Behavioral/emotional problems in mentally retarded children and youth. *Psychol Rep* **51**, 143–146.

Hagerman RJ (1996) Physical and behavioral phenotype. In: Hagerman RJ, Cronister AC (eds) *Fragile X Syndrome: Diagnosis, Treatment and Research*. Baltimore: Johns Hopkins University Press, pp.3–87.

Hagerman RJ, Cronister AC (eds) *Fragile X Syndrome: Diagnosis, Treatment and Research*. Baltimore: Johns Hopkins University Press.

Hall S, Oliver C, Murphy G (2001) Self-injurious behaviour in young children with Lesch–Nyhan syndrome. *Dev Med Child Neurol* **43**, 745–749.

Hatton C (1998) Intellectual disabilities – epidemiology and causes. In: Emerson E, Hatton C, Bromley J, Caine A (eds) *Clinical Psychology and People with Intellectual Disabilities*. Chichester: Wiley.

Hollins S, Esterhuyzen A (1997) Bereavement and grief in adults with learning disabilities. *Br J Psychiatr* **170**, 497–501.

Howlin P (2000) Autism and intellectual disability: diagnostic and treatment issues. *J Roy Soc Med* **93**, 351–355.

Ishii T, Takahashi O, Kawamura Y, Ohta T (2003) Comorbidity in attention deficit-hyperactivity disorder. *Psychiatr Clin Neurosci* **57**, 457–463.

Jansen DE, Krol B, Groothoff JW, Post D (2004) People with intellectual disability and their health problems: a review of comparative studies. *J Intellect Disabil Res* **48**, 93–102.

Jyothy A, Rao GN, Kumar KS, et al. (2002) Translocation Down syndrome. *Indian J Med Sci* **56**, 225–229.

Kent L, Evans J, Paul M, Sharp M (1999) Comorbidity of autistic spectrum disorders in children with Down syndrome. *Dev Med Child Neurol* **41**, 153–158.

Koller H, Richardson SA, Katz M, Mclaren J (1983) Behavior disturbance since childhood among a 5-year birth cohort of all mentally retarded young adults in a city. *Am J Mental Defic* **87**, 386–395.

Koning C, Magill-Evans J (2001) Social and language skills in adolescent boys with Asperger syndrome. *Autism* **5**, 23–36.

Lee KT, Mattson SN, Riley EP (2004) Classifying children with heavy prenatal alcohol exposure using measures of attention. *J Int Neuropsychol Soc* **10**, 271–277.

Loesch DZ, Bui QM, Grigsby J, et al. (2003) Effect of the fragile X status categories and the fragile X mental retardation protein levels on executive functioning in males and females with fragile X. *Neuropsychology* **17**, 646–657.

Lorenz S (1998) *Children with Down's Syndrome: A Guide for Teachers and Support Assistants in Mainstream Education*. London: David Fulton.

Marder EM, Dennis J (2001) Medical management of children with Down's syndrome. *Curr Paediatr* **11**, 57–63.

May C, Male I, Mills A, Turk J (2003) Is there a FraX-E phenotype? A systematic review. Paper presented at the Royal College of Paediatrics and Child Health Annual Meeting, University of York. London: Royal College of Paediatrics and Child Health.

McClintock K, Hall S, Oliver C (2003) Risk markers associated with challenging behaviours in people with intellectual disabilities: a meta-analytic study. *J Intellect Disabil Res* **47**, 405–416.

Merritt L (2003) Recognition of the clinical signs and symptoms of Joubert syndrome. *Adv Neonat Care* **3**, 178–186.

Metcalfe K (1999) Williams syndrome: an update on clinical and molecular aspects. *Arch Dis Child* **81**, 198–199.

Nordin V, Gillberg C (1996) Autism spectrum disorders in children with physical or mental disability or both. I: Clinical and epidemiological aspects. *Dev Med Child Neurol* **38**, 297–313.

O'Brien G (2002) *Behavioural Phenotypes in Clinical Practice*. London: Mac Keith Press.

Oliver C (1995) Annotation: self-injurious behaviour in children with learning disabilities: recent advances in assessment and intervention. *J Child Psychol Psychiatr* **30**, 909–927.

Oliver C, Murphy G, Hall S, Arron K, Leggett J (2003) Phenomenology of self-restraint. *Am J Mental Retard* **108**, 71–81.

Philips I, Williams N (1975) Psychopathology and mental retardation: a study of 100 mentally retarded children: I. psychopathology. *Am J Psychiatr* **132**, 1265–1271.

Plomin R (1988). *Nature and Nurture: Introduction to Human Behavioural Genetics*. Florence, KY: Brooks Cole.

Rasmussen P, Börjesson O, Wentz E, Gillberg C (2001) Autistic disorders in Down syndrome: background factors and clinical correlates. *Dev Med Child Neurol* **43,** 750–754.

Reif A, Lesch KP (2003) Toward a molecular architecture of personality. *Behav Brain Res* **139**, 1–20.

Robey KL, Reck JF, Giacomini KD, Barabas G, Eddey GE (2003) Modes and patterns of self-mutilation in persons with Lesch–Nyhan disease. *Dev Med Child Neurol* **45**, 167–171.

Rogers, S.J., Hepburn, S.L., Stackhouse, T. & Wehner, E. (2003). Imitation performance in toddlers with autism and those with other developmental disorders. *Journal of Child Psychology & Psychiatry*, **44**, 763–781.

Rutter M, Graham P, Yule W (1970) *A Neuropsychiatric Study in Childhood*. London: Heinemann.

Scarr S, McCartney K (1983) How people make their own environments: a theory of genotype greater than environment effects. *Child Dev* **54**, 424–435.

Selikowitz M (1997). *Down's Syndrome – The Facts.* Oxford: Oxford University Press.

Smith AC Dykens E, Greenberg F (1998) Behavioral phenotype of Smith–Magenis syndrome (del 17p11.2). *Am J Med Genet* **81**, 179–185.

Soderstrom H, Rastam M, Gillberg C (2002) Temperament and character in adults with Asperger syndrome. *Autism* **6**, 287–297.

Steffenburg S, Gillberg C, Steffenburg U (1996) Psychiatric disorders in children and adolescents with mental retardation and active epilepsy. *Arch Neurol* **53**, 904–912.

Symons FJ, Clark RD, Hatton DD, Skinner M, Bailey DB (2003) Self-injurious behaviour in young boys with fragile X syndrome. *Am J Med Genet* **118A**, 115–121.

Tarjan I, Balaton G, Balaton P, Varbiro S, Vajo Z (2003) Facial and dental appearance of Williams syndrome. *Postgrad Med J* **79**, 241.

Taylor C (2004) Speech and language therapy. In: Dew-Hughes D (ed) *Educating Children with Fragile X Syndrome*. London: Routledge Falmer, pp.106–114.

Turk J (1996) Working with parents of children who have severe learning disabilities. *Clin Child Psychol Psychiatr* **1**, 581–596.

Turk J (1997) The mental health needs of children with learning disabilities. In: Holt G, Kon Y, Bouras N (eds) *Mental Health in Learning Disabilities, Training Package*. Brighton: Pavillion Publications.

Turk J (1998) Fragile X syndrome and attentional deficits. *J Appl Res Intellect Disabil* **11**, 175–191.

Turk J, Cornish KM (1998) Face recognition and emotion perception in boys with fragile-X syndrome. *J Intellect Disabil Res* **42**, 490–499.

Turk J, Graham P (1997) Fragile X syndrome, autism and autistic features. *Autism* **1**, 175–197.

Turk J, Patton M (2000) Sensory impairment and head circumference in fragile X syndrome, Down syndrome and idiopathic intellectual disability. *J Intellect Dev Disabil* **25**, 59–68.

Turk J, Das D, Howlin P, Barber N, Mottaleb M (2003) A follow-up study of intellectual, social and communicatory functioning in boys and young men with fragile X syndrome. Paper presented at the Society for the Study of Behavioural Phenotypes 10th Annual Scientific Meeting, Newcastle. Cambridge: Society for the Study of Behavioural Phenotypes.

Turk V, Brown H (1993) The sexual abuse of adults with learning disabilities: results of a two year incidence survey. *Mental Handicap Res* **6**, 193–216.

Turk J, Bax M, Williams C, Amin P, Eriksson M, Gillberg C (2009) Autism Spectrum Disorder in Children with and without Epilepsy: Impact on Social Functioning and Communication. *Acta Paediatrica Scandinavia* **98**, 675–681.

Turk J, Graham PJ, Verhulst F (2007) *Child & Adolescent Psychiatry: A Developmental Approach (4th edition)*. Oxford: Oxford University Press.

Van Borsel J, Curfs LM, Fryns JP (1997) Hyperacusis in Williams syndrome: a sample survey study. *Genet Counsel* **8**, 121–126.

Veltman MW, Thompson RJ, Roberts SE, Thomas NS, Whittington J, Bolton PF (2004) Prader–Willi syndrome – a study comparing deletion and uniparental disomy cases with reference to autism spectrum disorders. *Eur J Child Adolesc Psychiatr* **3**, 42–50.

Waters J (1999) *Prader–Willi Syndrome: A Practical Guide*. London: David Fulton.

Wing L, Gould J (1979) Severe impairments of social interaction and associated abnormalities in children: epidemiology and classification. *J Autism Dev Disord* **9**, 11–29.

World Health Organization (1992) *The ICD-10 Classification of Mental and Behavioural Disorders: Clinical Descriptions and Diagnostic Guidelines*. Geneva: World Health Organization.

2
HETEROGENEITY IN CEREBRAL PALSY: VARIATIONS IN NEUROLOGY, COMORBIDITY AND ASSOCIATED CONDITIONS

J Keith Brown and Paul Eunson

Introduction

In the 19th century, it was taught 'know syphilis, know clinical medicine'. The equivalent in this century would be 'know cerebral palsy, know clinical neurology'. Virtually all clinical signs can be found in studying cerebral palsy, and there are some such as subcortical reflex function which are rarely seen in other clinical situations. When children are examined, no two children are identical, as there is considerable variation even within a commonly described topographical syndrome such as hemiplegia. The variation in complications such as hip dislocation, scoliosis and gastrointestinal (GI) motor disorders is marked.

We shall consider as comorbidity any condition which is associated with the index condition, and which can appear as an *individual* entity in its own right in other patients. The difficulty in child neurology is that many of the major conditions, e.g. intellectual disability, epilepsy, cerebral palsy, attention-deficit and hyperkinetic disorder, autism, are not disease entities but syndromes. As all these conditions arise from brain dysfunction, they can occur in isolation, in any combination or together.

Symptom complexes or syndromes are a collection of clinical signs and symptoms which cluster, are not disease entities and have many aetiologies. When planning clinical services, this syndromic approach is valuable as the differing syndromes will require different interventions to manage the condition, although curing the primary cause is not possible. If services for children with these syndromes as a result of brain dysfunction work closely together, then the situation where each is viewed as a distinct disease entity can be avoided.

Terminology

Different societies have different preferences for how to describe developmental difficulties, particularly learning difficulties. Some medical terms have a derogatory meaning for the public. 'Spastic' as an adjective or noun to describe a child can be viewed as insulting, yet the term 'spasticity' remains a very useful word to describe a particular type of muscle hypertonus. A commonly used phrase such as 'autistic tendencies' or 'on the autistic spectrum' may confuse rather than illuminate the child's problems, and it would be preferable to describe the child's specific difficulties.

Brain syndromes

It is not surprising that if we select a group of children with brain damage on the basis of one function, i.e. motor dysfunction, then we find a whole spectrum of associated brain dysfunctions in association with the index disorder – cerebral palsy.

Cerebral palsy can occur in conjunction with the following.

1. Epilepsy
2. Global cognitive learning disorder (intellectual disability)
3. Specific cognitive learning disorder:
    a. Specific language impairment
    b. Dyslexia
    c. Dyscalculia
    d. Spelling dysgraphia
4. Dysgraphia
5. Peripheral and central deafness
6. Speech and language disorder:
    a. Slow speech development
    b. Dysarthria
7. Autism
8. Attention-deficit disorder
9. Visual impairment:
    a. Blindness
    b. Visual field defects
    c. Squints
    d. Myopia
    e. Specific visuospatial disorder
    f. Cerebral visual impairment
10. Stereotypies
11. Disordered fight and flight responses
12. Sudden death

These conditions are not caused by the cerebral palsy, are not complications of the cerebral palsy but are comorbid. As they are caused by the same aetiology, they are also cocausal. The frequencies of these cocausal conditions vary with the cause and the type of cerebral palsy but broadly are as follows.

1. Epilepsy   31–44% (Shevell et al. 2009)
2. Global learning disorder   46% (Schenker et al. 2005)
3. Speech disorders   28% (Schenker et al. 2005)

4. Behaviour disorder   25% (Carlsson et al. 2008, Parkes et al. 2008)
5. Specific learning difficulties   36% (Frampton et al. 1998)
6. Abnormal visual perception   70% (Guzzetta et al. 2001)

This broad spectrum of comorbid conditions determines the holistic assessment of the child in the home, school and community by a range of therapists.

1. Posture and mobility
2. Manipulation
3. Visuospatial development
4. Hearing
5. Speech and language, communication and understanding
6. Non-verbal communication
7. Feeding, nutrition and growth
8. Behaviour, social and emotional development
9. Activities of daily living, personal and social independence
10. Epilepsy
11. Education – specific and global learning abilities
12. Musical abilities

There is a group of complications seen more frequently in children suffering from cerebral palsy which give rise to conditions which in other circumstances can be seen as disorders in their own right.

1. Umbilical hernia
2. Inguinal hernia
3. High arched palate
4. Swallowing difficulties
5. Gastro-oesophageal reflux
6. Constipation
7. Anaemia
8. Malnutrition
9. Growth failure
10. Dislocated hips
11. Windswept posture of legs and pelvis
12. Scoliosis
13. Osteoporosis
14. Recurrent fractures
15. Joint contractures
16. Aspiration pneumonia
17. Haemangiomata
18. Plagiocephaly
19. Microcephaly
20. Macrocephaly

The complications involving gastrointestinal motor function, from disorders of chewing and swallowing to reflux, disordered stomach motility and constipation, have similarities to the upper motor neurone lesions affecting skeletal muscle in cerebral palsy – weakness, poor co-ordination, poor fine motor skills, exaggerated reflexes as well as disordered sensation – and may be considered as an autonomic motor syndrome.

However, and here is the confusion, a non-motor problem seen more commonly than chance in cerebral palsy can be comorbid, cocausal or a complication. For example, epilepsy in association with cerebral palsy can be:

- *Comorbid* – familial childhood absence epilepsy
- *Cocausal* – secondary to antenatal middle cerebral artery infarct
- *Complication* – secondary to anoxia injury after aspiration pneumonia.

Until you look at the aetiology in detail, it may not be clear what the relationship is between cerebral palsy and accompanying non-motor conditions. This is particularly the case with learning difficulties, both specific and global.

Neurological heterogeneity and cerebral palsy
Cerebral palsy is a motor disorder affecting movements and posture due to damage to the developing brain. Bax's definition has stood the test of time and has been used for epidemiological studies – a non-progressive disorder of movement and posture due to a defect or lesion of the immature brain (Bax 1964). More recently a working party (Rosenbaum et al. 2006) has proposed an expanded definition which acknowledges the functional implications of the disorder and the frequency of accompanying disturbances: "Cerebral palsy (CP) describes a group of permanent disorders of the development of movement and posture, causing activity limitation, that are attributed to nonprogressive disturbances that occurred in the developing fetal or infant brain. The motor disorders of cerebral palsy are often accompanied by disturbances of sensation, perception, cognition, communication, and behaviour; by epilepsy, and by secondary musculoskeletal problems." The clinical disorder of posture and movement does change with time and brain development and may appear to get functionally worse. However, the cause is non-progressive.

Cerebral palsy forms one of a group of conditions affecting mobility in children, resulting in a chronic physical disability.

1. *Orthopaedic disorders* – congenital dislocation of the hip, juvenile rheumatoid arthritis, obstetric brachial plexus injuries, amputees, land mine injuries
2. *Muscle disorders* – muscular dystrophies, myopathies, inflammatory muscle diseases
3. *Spinal disorders* – spina bifida, spinal muscular atrophy, poliomyelitis, spinal trauma
4. *Cerebral disorders* – any chronic motor disorder arising from brain damage, including damage from genetic causes

The delay in acquiring motor skills does not follow the severity of spasticity or presence of abnormal neurological findings (Figure 2.1). Some children with alarming choreo-athetosis will walk and rarely fall. Neurological examination of a child with hemiplegia will not tell you whether he or she will walk at 1 year or 4 years. The child may have bilateral brisk reflexes, ankle clonus and extensor plantar response but walk well.

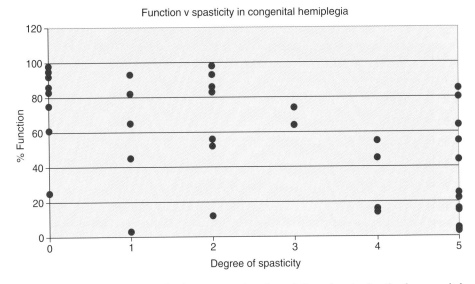

Figure 2.1 Lack of close correlation between severity of spasticity and motor function in congenital hemiplegia.

Many interventions have been used in the past in an attempt to manage the motor disorder in children with cerebral palsy, yet only recently has there been focus on improving function, particularly using the Gross Motor Function Measure (Palisano et al. 2000) as an assessment tool. A delay of greater than 2 standard deviations below the mean in an aspect of motor function should be included in a definition for cerebral palsy. Children with lesser degrees of motor delay are not without some degree of functional limitation. Although they may walk, they may have difficulty in acquiring more sophisticated motor skills, such as running, jumping, swimming or playing ball games.

WHAT CONSTITUTES MOTOR FUNCTION?
Normal motor function can be divided into several functional divisions.

- Posture
- Mobility
- Hand function
- Bulbar function
  - Bite
  - Chew
  - Swallow
- Eye movements
- Emotional motor function
- Autonomic motor function

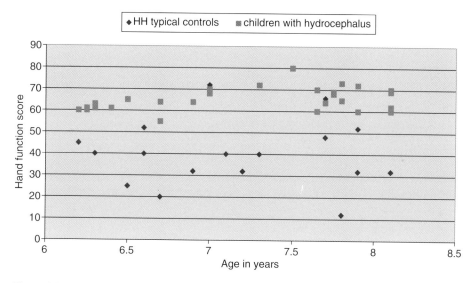

Figure 2.2 Comparison of hand function between children with hydrocephalus and typical controls.

The term 'cerebral palsy' is normally restricted to abnormal posture and mobility even though abnormal eye movements, bulbar dysfunction and autonomic dysfunction frequently coexist. Dyspraxia, bulbar palsy or gastrointestinal motor disorders may exist in isolation. If occurring along with cerebral palsy, should they be considered comorbid, cocausal, a complication or should the cerebral palsy syndrome be expanded to encompass these motor phenomena? Hydrocephalus and its sequelae after shunting can have a significant impact on motor function – gross motor, fine motor (Figure 2.2), bulbar function, prosody – but without necessarily producing upper motor neurone signs.

CLASSIFICATION OF CEREBRAL PALSY

A detailed discussion of the classification of cerebral palsy by topographical distribution, tone abnormality, severity and aetiology is not relevant in this chapter. The importance of classifying the type of cerebral palsy is that it guides the clinician and therapist to what comorbid conditions and complications are more likely to be present in the individual child, e.g.:

- child who does not bear weight– dislocated hips
- diplegia associated with preterm birth – specific intellectual disability
- middle cerebral artery infarct – visual field defect
- ataxic cerebral palsy – intellectual disability and epilepsy.

With the advent of magnetic resonance imaging (MRI), the clinician now has a clearer picture of underlying aetiology and the sequence of events that led to the brain damage, particularly if this is a complication of preterm labour, preterm birth or term hypoxic ischaemic encephalopathy. This information also assists in predicting non-motor developmental delay in the individual child.

Box 2.1 Non-motor symptoms and signs in hemiplegic cerebral palsy

- Mean IQ 100
  - Mean IQ 85 if epilepsy present
- Normal bladder and bowel control
- Attention-deficit–hyperactivity disorder 5%
  - 33% if epilepsy present
- Scoliosis rare except with significant leg length discrepancy

---

- Profound brief hypoxia – basal ganglia lesion – dystonic cerebral palsy + normal intellect
- Subacute chronic hypoxia – watershed infarcts – quadriplegic cerebral palsy, epilepsy and intellectual disabilities

Classifying by severity predicts deformity which is a consequence of the immobility rather than the neurological deficit. The child who is unable to walk or bear weight is much more at risk of hip dislocation and subsequent asymmetrical sitting posture. In many children this leads inevitably to windswept posture and to kyphoscoliosis, despite good positioning programmes. Deformities can be postural, due to abnormal muscle tone, or positional, due to effects of gravity and positioning. The two often work in tandem.

A strictly unilateral lesion does not affect trunk or neck muscles, rarely affects bulbar function and does not affect bowel or bladder function. Therefore the child with hemiplegic cerebral palsy should not develop scoliosis, should not be at risk of aspiration pneumonia and should develop continence. Virtually all children with hemiplegic cerebral palsy will walk, unless there is associated severe intellectual disability. The exception to this is the child who has a unilateral motor lesion but bilateral brain damage, e.g. asymmetrical periventricular leucomalacia, who is at risk of the non-motor symptoms associated with diplegic or quadriplegic cerebral palsy (Box 2.1).

However, there is considerable variation in motor signs, particularly if one considers hand position (Figure 2.3). This will be a manifestation of the underlying structural injury – position and size – and impact of therapy.

The child with bilateral lesions in the brain will usually have a diplegic or quadriplegic pattern of cerebral palsy, although differentiating these two entities is difficult as they do share motor and non-motor features (Box 2.2). Quadriplegic cerebral palsy is more than just a bilateral hemiplegia as the midline structures are involved, and the risks of global intellectual disability, epilepsy, visual impairment and bulbar dysfunction are much higher.

Epilepsy in quadriplegic cerebral palsy is more likely to be intractable and to start in the first year of life in comparison with other geographical subtypes of cerebral palsy. The motor signs in quadriplegic cerebral palsy vary from child to child and may change in the same child with time and therapy. The presence or absence of dystonia and other

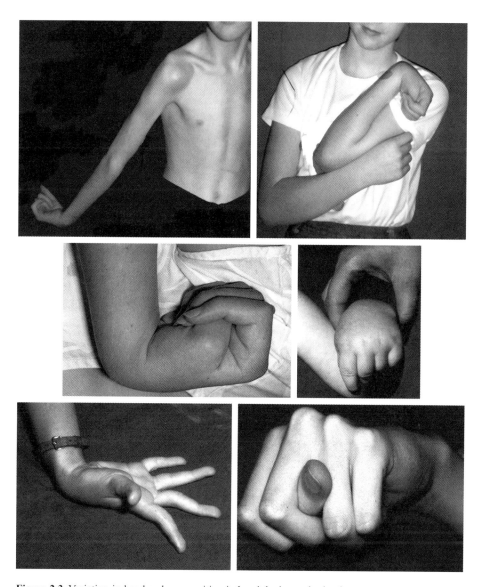

Figure 2.3 Variation in hand and arm position in hemiplegic cerebral palsy.

extrapyramidal factors influences the position of the child at rest (Figure 2.4) and with attempted movement.

The child who has a diplegic cerebral palsy as a result of preterm birth has the additional risks of complications of preterm birth which are not a direct consequence of acquired brain damage or cerebral palsy (Box 2.3). Teasing out which are comorbid, which are cocausal and which are complications of cerebral palsy is probably not essential for managing the problem, but is critical for preventing it.

Box 2.2 Non-motor symptoms and signs in 21 children with severe quadriplegic cerebral palsy (Brown & Minns 1998)

Gastrointestinal and nutrition
Hiatus hernia	28%
Reflux oesophagitis	33%
Nasogastric feeding	28%
Constipation	76%
Growth failure	52%
Anaemia	10%

Respiratory
Recurrent aspirations	19%
Recurrent chest infections	14%

Continence
Most incontinent with no bladder or bowel control

Orthopaedic
Contractures	47%
Dislocated hips common	
Scoliosis/windswept	66%

Intellectual and communication
Intellectual disability	90%
Most no speech	
Epilepsy	60–76%

Specific learning difficulties are frequently found in children with diplegic cerebral palsy. Visuospatial difficulties are well recognised and in themselves do not adversely affect a child's performance in school overall. However, children with cerebral palsy may also have difficulties in working memory and executive function (Jenks et al. 2009) and struggle to cope with education in a mainstream setting.

A pure dystonic cerebral palsy as a result of a hypoxic injury to the basal ganglia in the term infant produces a bilateral motor disorder which may be profound – the child has a severe motor dyspraxia affecting hand and leg function, bulbar function and speech production. The dystonic spasms may be painful, and accompanying dykinesia may be so severe that the child fails to grow through an inability to take in sufficient calories to compensate for increased basal metabolic rate. However, intellect may be preserved, and if the child is

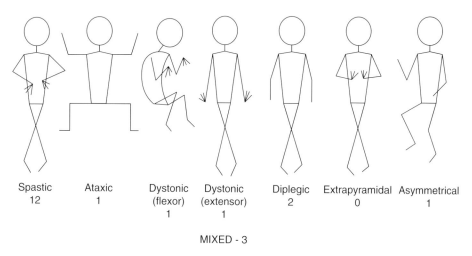

Spastic	Ataxic	Dystonic	Dystonic	Diplegic	Extrapyramidal	Asymmetrical
12	1	(flexor)	(extensor)	2	0	1
		1	1			

MIXED - 3

Figure 2.4 Neurological type of quadriplegic cerebral palsy determines position at rest.

Box 2.3 Non-motor signs and symptoms in diplegic cerebral palsy

- Epilepsy 34% (Himmelmann et al. 2006)
  - High if low Apgar + perinatal asphyxia
- Intelligence quotient – 68–98 interquartile range (Sigurdardottir et al. 2008)
- Specific intellectual disabilities (Bowen et al. 2002, Schenker et al. 2005)
  - Dyslexia
  - Dysgraphia
  - Arithmetic difficulties
  - Upper limb dyspraxia

---

provided with appropriate augmented communication methods, the child's quality of life can improve immensely. Epilepsy and visual impairment are unusual in this group.

Magnetic resonance imaging studies in populations of children with cerebral palsy have helped to explain some of the heterogeneity of the motor abnormalities (Table 2.1). This also can explain the variation in the presence of comorbid/cocausal conditions – for example, in hemiplegic cerebral palsy:

- MRI middle cerebral artery infarct – risk of epilepsy high
- MRI internal capsule lesion – risk of epilepsy negligible.

What explanations can be postulated for the heterogeneity in neurological features, the variations in other developmental disorders and the frequency of complications in cerebral palsy?

TABLE 2.1
MRI findings in the European Cerebral Palsy Study by
topographical distribution (Bax et al. 2006)

	N	%
Periventricular brain tissue loss	147	42
Basal ganglia damage	44	12.6
Cortical/subcortical damage	33	9.4
Focal cortical infarcts	26	7.4
Malformation	31	8.9
Normal imaging	44	12.6
Miscellaneous	25	7.1

1. Risk factors
2. Age of fetus at time of lesion
3. Gestation at birth
4. Complications of prematurity
5. Complications of prolonged neonatal intensive care
6. Effects of interventions
7. Access to therapy
8. Age of child at assessment
9. Epilepsy
10. Nutrition

RISK FACTORS
Genetic, maternal, intrauterine and socio-economic factors have the potential for predisposing the child to cerebral palsy and independently to other childhood disorders, i.e. comorbid disorders. Single-gene causes of cerebral palsy are rare but are associated with severe intellectual disability. Intrauterine growth retardation is a risk factor for cerebral palsy (Jacobsson et al. 2008) but is also associated with developmental delay and poor school performance in the absence of a motor impairment. Maternal malnutrition puts the child at risk of obstructed labour (Konje & Ladipo 2000) with associated risk of obstetric brain damage and is also independently a cause of intellectual problems in school.

AGE OF FETUS AT TIME OF LESION
Insults to the brain of a fetus in the first trimester may result in fetal death and spontaneous miscarriage. In the second trimester, the brain is undergoing rapid development and an insult may result in migration abnormalities or cessation of brain growth. In the second and third trimesters, between 24 and 32 weeks, the developing white matter is particularly at risk. Preterm labour may ensue or be induced, and the child then is at risk of the complications of preterm birth. The basal ganglia in the term infant are highly sensitive to the toxic effects of bilirubin.

Therefore, depending on the maturity of the brain, similar insults will have different effects. Depending on stage of development and maturity of other organs, the insult may affect their function in different ways, and some of the non-motor disorders associated with cerebral palsy may be the result of ischaemic or toxic injuries to other organs at critical stages of their development.

GESTATION AT BIRTH

Cooke & Abernethy (1999) studied 87 very-low-birthweight (VLBW) infants and eight term controls who had been examined psychometrically at school between the ages of 12 and 13 years, and had cranial MRI at 15–17 years of age. No significant differences in intelligence quotient, motor clumsiness or frequency of attention-deficit–hyperactivity disorder were observed between those children with MRI lesions and those with normal scans. Thirty seven of the total 87 (42.5%) VLBW children had abnormalities reported on their scans. These were the typical white matter pathology of low birthweight – two porencephaly, 28 periventricular leucomalacia, 24 ventricular dilation, five thinning of the corpus callosum). This study illustrates how some comorbidities such as intellectual and behaviour disorders do not follow the pathology of the motor defect, i.e. periventricular leucomalacia with spastic diplegia (see later), but are independent variables due to prematurity.

The child born very preterm is at risk of a brain insult around the time of birth, and remains vulnerable for some weeks to further insults not directly caused by the initial insult, for example, a period of hypotension related to a respiratory event. Signs and symptoms may arise from the second episode, adding to heterogeneity. Is this a comorbid condition? The presence or absence of hydrocephalus after an intraventricular haemorrhage alters the child's developmental prognosis. If the hydrocephalus arises late, is this complication, cocausal or comorbid?

COMPLICATIONS OF PRETERM BIRTH

The very preterm infant is at risk of respiratory disease, gastrointestinal disease, bone disease and eye disease which are not necessarily causally related to the event or events that resulted in the brain lesion. In later childhood, these disorders may contribute to the developmental problems presumed to be secondary to the brain lesion – for example, retinopathy of prematurity, posterior periventricular leucomalacia and cortical visual impairment may all coexist in the same child to affect vision profoundly.

Neurological and developmental outcomes of preterm birth include the following.

- Squints
- Vertical hemianopia
- Myopia
- Blindness
- Cerebral visual impairment
- Slow speech development
- Deafness
- Visuospatial problems

- Visuomotor problems
- Dyscalculia
- Slow motor learning/clumsy/manual dyspraxia
- Small stature
- Cerebral palsy

The majority of these signs and symptoms can be explained by the white matter damage. Short stature is probably multifactorial. Periventricular leucomalacia from events around 32 weeks' gestation is more likely to be posterior and can produce the complex visual problems without a motor disorder.

COMPLICATIONS OF PROLONGED NEONATAL INTENSIVE CARE

The neonate who has not been fed orally until a few months of age because of respiratory or GI disease may have great difficulty gaining oral feeding skills and have a severe oromotor dyspraxia and food aversion. This is presumed to be caused by the child being unable to practise these skills at a critical stage of development and being unable to develop central pattern generators that co-ordinate motor, sensory and respiratory functions to allow safe feeding.

Similarly, does prolonged neonatal intensive care interfere with mother–child bonding and cause an emotional dyspraxia in the child because of this separation at a crucial stage?

The child who has been born preterm, has had a neonatal hypoxic-ischaemic insult and has had the complications of preterm birth may therefore have suffered multiple insults at different stages of brain development (Box 2.4). MRI and other imaging modalities and electroencephalographs (EEG) may only hint at the range and severity of pathology (Figure 2.5).

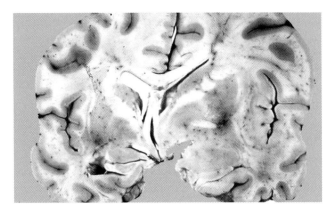

Figure 2.5 Subependymal haemorrhage, periventricular white matter damage and kernicterus in the same brain.

Box 2.4 Potential pathologies affecting brain of child born preterm

- Genetic disease syndrome
- Congenital brain malformation
- Antenatal maternal drug and alcohol misuse
- Subependymal/germinal layer haemorrhage
- Infarctive cystic periventricular leucomalacia
- Perinatal telencephalic leucoencephalopathy
- Secondary hydrocephalus and fourth ventricle hydrocephalus
- Traumatic brain damage from birth trauma
- Hypoxic ischaemic encephalopathy
- Hyperbilirubinaemic encephalopathy
- Thrombophilic primary vessel thrombosis (protein C & S, factor V Leiden)
- Intracerebral haemorrhage – clotting disorder
- Pontine necrosis

EFFECTS OF INTERVENTIONS

Survival and prevalence of cerebral palsy have been the measures of outcome commonly used in pregnancy and neonatal intensive care. Ideally, one should look at how well the young person is functioning as they enter adult life – motor, intellectual, social and emotional functioning. That is difficult as there are so many additional factors in childhood that may affect prognosis and it is difficult to maintain follow-up particularly in the child who is relatively well.

There are no standardised guidelines with good evidence base for types or frequency of therapy in children with cerebral palsy. Some physiotherapy philosophies use the child's abnormal muscle tone for functional tasks, other philosophies concentrate on normalising tone. In Britain, there is inequitable access to botulinum toxin therapy and intrathecal baclofen therapy. Educational provision for the child with a motor disorder may be in special school or in mainstream school.

Prevalence of cerebral palsy has not changed greatly in the last 30 years and with survival at the limits of viability better, there may be children with more severe neurological and other organ involvement surviving. When a new intervention in management of the preterm child is introduced, are we measuring all potential outcomes and is follow-up long enough?

Cooling of the infant with a severe hypoxic ischaemic encephalopathy and neonatal encephalopathy has been recently introduced and initial results are promising. Will this change the pattern of long term outcome for this group and will the improvement be across the spectrum – less epilepsy, fewer speech and language difficulties, less severe cerebral palsy?

The child may have limited access to therapy due to geography, health service resources or parental beliefs. It is difficult to argue strongly for some therapies as the evidence base is still lacking. Crudely, it is understood that not paying attention to positioning in the more severely affected child leads to earlier onset of contractures and deformities.

Deformities in children with cerebral palsy are often a result of the neurological deficit, i.e. due to one or more of the following:

- paresis with muscle imbalance
- abnormal sequencing of muscle action
- spasticity
- dystonic rigidity
- arrested muscle growth
- secondary biomechanical plastic change
- ataxia
- dyskinesia.

However, there are certain deformities in children with cerebral palsy which are not the result of the neurological deficit but are due to the immobility, the effects of gravity and the position in which the child is placed (Brown & Minns 1989). Deformity develops as a result of external forces acting on the body rather than internal deforming forces secondary to neurological damage. We have called these positional deformities since they depended upon the position in which the child was positioned or nursed (Brown 1985, Fulford & Brown 1976). They are not *postural* deformities as this suggests that they have a neurological basis, being due to an abnormal postural muscle tone or dystonia imposing a particular posture (Figure 2.6).

Attention focused too closely on the motor disorder, for example, may adversely affect a child's access to education and socialisation with ultimately a poorer outcome. Martin Bax (personal communication) was told by some young adults with cerebral palsy that he had paid too much attention to getting them to walk when they were children and they were never going to be able to walk. They would have preferred more time to be spent on their communication skills and controlling their drooling of saliva.

AGE OF CHILD AT ASSESSMENT

Until a child reaches the age at which they could be expected to attain a skill, this morbidity cannot be diagnosed. It can be anticipated if the initiating event is well understood. Hemiplegic cerebral palsy is often not diagnosed until 6 months of age when it is apparent that the child is not developing skills in one arm and the hand on that side remains fisted and flexed at the elbow. The more subtle intellectual disabilities associated with periventricular leucomalacia are not detected until a child is into school.

A child with diplegic cerebral palsy may develop household mobility and some community mobility in the first decade of life with the aid of orthoses and walking frames or sticks. However, the child never gets to the stage of having good community mobility, and is unable to take part in sport upon their feet. Then, with increase in weight and progression of muscle shortening, particularly of the hamstrings and hip flexors (Figure 2.7), the energy

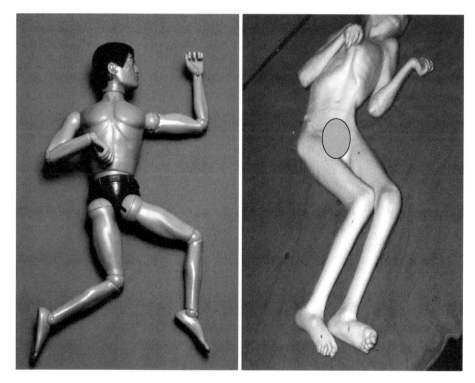

Figure 2.6 Positional deformities.

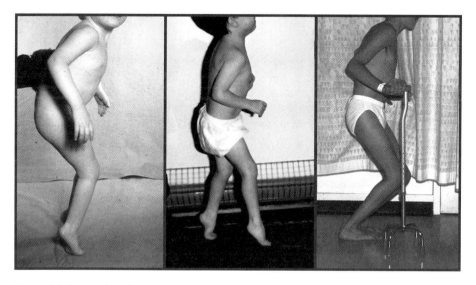

Figure 2.7 Progression of contractures in diplegic cerebral palsy with age.

required to continue walking is too great and the child, now a teenager, reverts to wheelchair use. The pathology is static, the effects progress.

EPILEPSY

Epilepsy following an ischaemic injury to the brain at birth can present at any stage from the neonatal period through to some months or years later, despite the child having had seizures and an abnormal EEG at the time of the severe neonatal encephalopathy. The type and severity of the seizure disorder will vary with the brain lesion. In children who subsequently develop quadriplegic cerebral palsy with severe cognitive difficulties, the epilepsy may be intractable and initially present as infantile spasms.

There is a particular age-dependent epilepsy type which is more common in hemiplegic cerebral palsy – electrical status epilepticus in sleep (ESES). It tends to develop between the ages of 5 and 10 years. The seizures may be relatively infrequent but when the child goes off to sleep, the EEG shows persistent spike wave discharge virtually throughout sleep but with no apparent clinical accompaniment. The status may be generalised or partial. The child may present with onset of language difficulties, poor school performance and cognitive decline. ESES tends to resolve spontaneously in the second decade and is rarely seen in adult life. However, it may interfere with learning during a critical stage in the child's education.

NUTRITION

Nutrition and growth in cerebral palsy is a complex subject with a number of interactions.

- Gene disorders or genetic risk factors may affect growth and cause cerebral palsy independently.
- The brain damage may affect hypothalamic and pituitary control of growth and cause cerebral palsy.
- The child may have a pseudobulbar palsy which affects calorie intake.
- The child may have coexisting disease which affects growth, e.g. short gut syndrome.
- The child may have a severe dyskinetic cerebral palsy where calorie intake cannot compensate for the increased energy expenditure of the involuntary movements.
- The child may have hypothalamic dysfunction which enhances growth, more often seen in the presence of profound disability.
- The child may be inappropriately fed, particularly through gastrostomy.
- Historically, infants born preterm were fed artificial milks deficient in essential fatty acids which affected myelination.
- Preterm infants and those with gastro-oesophageal reflux are at risk of iron deficiency anaemia which can have an adverse effect on gross motor development.
- In areas of the world where the soil is deficient in iodine, maternal iodine deficiency is associated with an increased risk of cerebral palsy, and iodine deficiency in the child is a risk factor for intellectual disability.
- The child born preterm is at risk of rickets of prematurity unless give adequate calcium and vitamin D supplements. If allowed to develop, the rickets will adversely affect bone

growth and modelling. If the child is subsequently non-weight bearing as a result of cerebral palsy, they may be at risk of osteoporosis with an additional risk of bone deformity.

Pervasive developmental disorders and cerebral palsy
Many of the comorbidities and complications described above can be linked directly or indirectly to the same brain damage that caused the cerebral palsy. Pervasive developmental disorders (PDD) and in particular classic autism occurring without the context of cerebral palsy are not associated with structural malformations of the brain or brain damage. The strongest risk factor for autism is to have a first-degree relative with autism. If a child with cerebral palsy meets the criteria for classic autism, this could be a true comorbidity. There are a number of possible processes by which the two apparently separate conditions could occur in the same child.

- There are a number of genetic diplegic and quadriplegic syndromes with varying accompanying features such as intellectual disability. The gene defect may code for the motor disorder and PDD.
- Pervasive developmental disorder is associated with obstetric complications which in turn may be a risk factor for cerebral palsy.
- The motor disability may affect the child's ability to participate in social life, hence adversely affecting communication skills.
- Visual deficits are common in cerebral palsy and children with impaired vision are more at risk of having PDD.
- Epilepsy and intellectual disability are risk factors for PDD and are more commonly found in children with cerebral palsy than their able-bodied peer group.

Pervasive developmental disorders are more common in children with cerebral palsy, 3–11% of children with cerebral palsy in two studies being given a diagnosis of autism (Goodman & Graham 1996, Kilinclasan & Mukaddes 2009). Autism with cerebral palsy was more common with more severe motor impairment, and in the presence of epilepsy, intellectual disability and speech disorders. This would suggest that the autism is more likely with more extensive brain damage, and therefore can be explained predominantly by the brain damage. Genetic factors are probably of less significance in the pathogenesis of PDD in a child with cerebral palsy than in a child with no other developmental disorder.

Conclusions
- Children with cerebral palsy have been traditionally described on the basis of tone abnormality, topographical distribution of motor impairment, and severity. All of these descriptors can change with time and the influence of therapy.
- Each topographical type of cerebral palsy has many causes.
- Each damaging process causing cerebral palsy can cause different topographical types.
- The brain injury or maldevelopment may affect all aspects of neurological function – the motor disorder is obvious at an earlier age than for example speech, yet the motor disorder may be relatively unimportant for determining quality of life in adult years.

- Infants born preterm are at risk of different insults to the brain occurring at different times.
- MRI of the brain will assist in determining what type of damaging event has occurred and when it occurred. This can help in predicting outcome and non-motor developmental difficulties.
- Neurological and developmental examination of the child will show an evolving process and should be used to determine changing priorities for therapy.
- All children with cerebral palsy deserve holistic assessment at appropriate developmental stages to identify the subtle disorders that may impinge on participation in society, particularly school.
- There are ongoing factors, particularly in quadriplegic cerebral palsy, which may adversely affect development, e.g. malnutrition, epilepsy, recurrent chest infections.
- Deciding if an accompanying disorder is comorbid, cocausal or a complication is not essential except for interventions designed to prevent such disorders. The child would prefer you to identify the disorder and decide what to do about it.

The future

The epidemiology of cerebral palsy and accompanying disorders will continue to change. With improvement in survival of children with severe forms of cerebral palsy, there is an increasing number coming to surgery for kyphoscoliosis and surviving into adult life. Assisted fertility with multiple births is a risk factor for cerebral palsy. Intracytoplasmic sperm injection has been associated with some malformations. Will this result in a new cohort of children with cerebral palsy and different comorbidities?

Follow-up of interventions to prevent or reduce the impact of antenatal, perinatal or postnatal brain damage must extend well into school age to allow assessment of learning, socialisation and behaviour.

Acknowledgement

Martin Bax contributed to the initial draft of this chapter.

REFERENCES

Bax M (1964) Terminology and classification of cerebral palsy. *Dev Med Child Neurol* **6**, 295–307.
Bax M, Tydeman C, Flodmark O (2006) Clinical and MRI correlates of cerebral palsy: the European Cerebral Palsy Study. *JAMA* **296(13)**, 1602–1608.
Bowen JR, Gibson FL, Hand PJ (2002) Educational outcome at 8 years for children who were born extremely prematurely: a controlled study. *J Paediatr Child Health* **38(5)**, 438–444.
Brown JK (1985) Positional deformity in children with cerebral palsy. *Physiother Pract* **1**, 37–41.
Brown JK, Minns RA (1989) Mechanism of deformity in children with cerebral palsy. *Semin Orthopaed* **14**, 236–255.
Brown JK, Minns RA (1998) Disorders of the central nervous system. In: Campbell A, McIntosh N (eds) Forfar and Arneil's Textbook of Paediatrics. Churchill Livingstone, Edinburgh, 1998.
Carlsson M, Olsson I, Hagberg G, et al. (2008) Behaviour in children with cerebral palsy with and without epilepsy. *Dev Med Child Neurol* **50(10)**, 784.
Cooke RW, Abernethy LJ (1999) Cranial magnetic resonance imaging and school performance in very low birth weight infants in adolescence. *Arch Dis Child Fetal Neonatal Ed* **81(2)**, 116–121.

Frampton I, Yude C, Goodman R (1998) The prevalence and correlates of specific learning difficulties in a representative sample of children with hemiplegia. *Br J Educ Psychol* **68(Pt 1)**, 39–51.

Fulford FE, Brown JK (1976) Position as a cause of deformity in children with cerebral palsy. *Dev Med Child Neurol* **18(3)**, 305–314.

Goodman R, Graham P (1996) Psychiatric problems in children with hemiplegia: cross sectional epidemiological survey. *BMJ* **312**, 1065–1069.

Guzzetta A, Mercuri E, Cioni G (2001) Visual disorder in children with brain lesion: 2. Visual impairment associated with cerebral palsy. *Eur J Paediatr Neurol* **5**, 115–119.

Himmelmann K, Beckung E, Hagberg G, et al. (2006) Gross and fine motor function and accompanying impairments in cerebral palsy. *Dev Med Child Neurol* **48(6)**, 417–423.

Jacobsson B, Ahlin K, Francis A, et al. (2008) Cerebral palsy and restricted growth status at birth: population-based case-control study. *Br J Obstet Gynaecol* **115(10)**, 1250–1255.

Jenks KM, de Moor J, van Lieshout E (2009) Arithmetic difficulties in children with cerebral palsy are related to executive function and working memory. *J Child Psychol Psychiatr* **50(7)**, 824–833.

Kilinclasan A, Mukaddes NM (2009) Pervasive developmental disorders in individuals with cerebral palsy. *Dev Med Child Neurol* **51(4)**, 289–294.

Konje JC, Ladipo OA (2000) Nutrition and obstructed labor. *Am J Clin Nutr* **72(1 Suppl)**, 291S–297S.

Palisano RJ, Hanna SE, Rosenbaum PL, et al. (2000) Validation of a model of gross motor function for children with cerebral palsy. *Phys Ther* **80(10)**, 974–985.

Parkes J, White-Koning M, Dickinson H (2008) Psychological problems in children with cerebral palsy: a cross-sectional European study. *J Child Psychol Psychiatr* **49(4)**, 405–413.

Rosenbaum P, Paneth N, Leviton A, Goldstein M, Bax M, Damiano D, Dan B, Jacobsson B (2006) The definition and classification of cerebral palsy. *Dev Med Child Neurol* **49(Suppl. 109)**, 8–14.

Schenker R, Coster WJ, Parush S (2005) Neuroimpairments, activity performance, and participation in children with cerebral palsy mainstreamed in elementary schools. *Dev Med Child Neurol* **47(12)**, 808–814.

Shevell MI, Dagenais L, Hall N, for the REPACQ Consortium (2009) Comorbidities in cerebral palsy and their relationship to neurologic subtype and GMFCS level. *Neurology* **72(24)**, 2090–2096.

Sigurdardottir S, Eiriksdottir A, Gunnarsdottir E, et al. (2008) Cognitive profile in young Icelandic children with cerebral palsy. *Dev Med Child Neurol* **50(5)**, 357–362.

Venkateswaran S, Shevell MI (2008) Comorbidities and clinical determinants of outcome in children with spastic quadriplegic cerebral palsy. *Dev Med Child Neurol* **50(3)**, 216–222.

3
GILLES DE LA TOURETTE SYNDROME AND ITS COMMON COMORBIDITIES

Michael Orth and Mary May Robertson

For well over a century after its first description by George Gilles de la Tourette, the syndrome that bears his name was considered a rare and exotic disease. This view has changed considerably. Epidemiological evidence suggests that Gilles de la Tourette syndrome (GTS) may be far more common than previously estimated, and it is now widely accepted that there is a significant genetic contribution to this neuropsychiatric disorder. However, despite the considerable advances in our understanding of GTS, the genetic basis of GTS remains elusive, the pathophysiology is incompletely understood and any interaction between genetic and potential environmental factors is speculative. From a clinical point of view, treating patients with GTS remains challenging because of the complexities of the clinical phenotype (Robertson 2000). In this chapter we will try to dissect, as much as is possible, GTS and its most frequent comorbidities, in particular attention-deficit–hyperactivity disorder (ADHD) and obsessive-compulsive disorder (OCD). This may help to improve the understanding of the trials and tribulations of patients with GTS; it also forms the basis of a systematic approach to assessment and treatment.

Symptoms and diagnosis of Gilles de la Tourette syndrome
Motor and phonic tics form the core symptoms of GTS. According to DSM-IV criteria, the diagnosis of GTS requires the presence of several motor and at least one phonic tic for more than 1 year. This distinguishes GTS from transient tics that can be observed as part of the normal development of children where they rarely last longer than 3–6 months, and from other tic disorders such as chronic motor or chronic phonic tics.

Tics can be defined as sudden, repetitive and stereotypical movements or sounds that involve discrete muscle groups (Leckman et al. 2001). Tics can be fast and brief with abrupt onset (clonic) or slow and sustained (tonic or dystonic), when they can resemble dystonia (Jankovic 1997). Tics can be simple (sudden, short and meaningless) or complex movements (prolonged, seemingly more purposeful). Examples of simple tics are eye blinking, nose twitching, head nodding, sniffing, throat clearing and coughing. Complex tics include often bizarre, complicated and socially embarrassing movements such as licking, smelling, spitting, jumping, twirling, touching (including another person's genitals) or noises including words and phrases such as 'that's it' or 'here we go', fluctuations of pitch and changing accents. The inappropriate uttering of expletives (coprolalia) represents the most readily identified complex phonic tic in GTS. While highly specific for GTS, it is important to note that the majority of patients, at least 70% in a specialist clinic and probably far more with mild GTS, do not have coprolalia (Robertson 1994). Other complex tics such as copropraxia (involuntary inappropriate obscene gestures), echolalia (imitation of sounds or words of others), echopraxia (imitation of actions of others), palilalia (repetition of one's own sounds or words) and palipraxia (repetition of one's own actions), as well as non-obscene complex socially inappropriate behaviours (NOSI, e.g. involuntary aspersions on a person's physical characteristics, such as weight or race (Kurlan et al. 1996)) also occur in a substantial proportion of patients with GTS.

The vast majority of patients report that tics are preceded by an inner feeling that is likened at times to an itch which needs to be relieved by the movement or noise (Bliss 1980, Leckman et al. 1993). Often patients battle to control these premonitory urges, e.g. to clear the throat or to shout or move; these feelings may be overwhelming and at times can be experienced as worse than the actual tic itself. These sensations are difficult to describe; they can refer to a particular anatomical region or may be a generalised inner tension that can only be relieved by a tic. In a highly individualised way, GTS patients also seem to be more sensitive to a variety of external perceptions, such as particular noises or words, but also shapes, rhythms or temperature changes, all of which can trigger both simple and complex tics. Patients are often able to suppress their tics for at least a short period of time unless tics are severe, in which case control may be greatly limited or even absent in the worst affected cases. Typically, stress and tiredness but sometimes relaxation and a comfortable environment can aggravate tics whereas distraction and, at times strikingly so, concentrating on a task may reduce the severity of tics.

Tics usually first arise between the ages of 3 and 8, and simple tics such as eye blinking are often the first to be observed. Phonic tics may also present as early as 3 years of age; however, they normally present later than motor tics. Tics usually occur in bouts in individual days and they wax and wane in intensity over weeks and months (Peterson & Leckman 1998). Tics often peak in their intensity at a mean age of about 10 (Leckman et al. 1998); thereafter, a considerable proportion of patients improve substantially in their teens, and may subjectively even consider themselves tic free, even though the expert eye may still detect tics (Leckman et al. 1998, Pappert et al. 2003).

Characteristically, over time patients acquire a repertoire of tics. Some tics are present at any given point in time before they disappear and are replaced by others.

At times it can be difficult to differentiate tics from other abnormal movements. These include stereotypies, myoclonus, chorea, dyskinesias and dystonia (Jankovic 2001). The age at onset of movements, presence or absence of premonitory sensations, the pattern of body regions involved and the temporal stability of symptoms but also comorbidities can give important clues to help differentiate tic disorders from other movement disorders. Premonitory urges, suppressibility and an inherent non-situational fluctuation of symptom severity over time, i.e. bouts of tics and waxing and waning, are essential characteristics of tics and are not features of other movement disorders. However, it needs to be borne in mind that some patients (e.g. young children or patients with intellectual disability) may find it difficult or even impossible to describe these features. Important differential diagnoses include benign childhood stereotypies, neuroacanthocytosis (where tics can be present but without

---

Box 3.1 Common comorbidities of GTS

- Disorders of inhibition and behaviour
  - Attention-deficit–hyperactivity disorder
  - Oppositional defiant disorder/conduct disorder
  - Rage attacks
- Obsessive-compulsive disorder and behaviours
- Mood disorders
  - Depression
  - Bipolar affective disorder
- Self-injurious behaviours
- Autistic spectrum disorders
- Others (e.g. dyslexia)

---

premonitory sensations or suppressibility), Wilson disease, Huntington disease, dystonia and psychogenic movement disorders (for further discussion see Jankovic 2001).

The comorbidities of Gilles de la Tourette syndrome

Gilles de la Tourette syndrome is often complicated by its comorbidities, in particular ADHD and OCD (Box 3.1). At least in a specialist interest clinic setting, one encounters more patients with comorbidities than patients who have 'pure', uncomplicated GTS. GTS may not be a single entity, with clinical (Freeman et al. 2000) and community studies (Khalifa & von Knorring 2005) suggesting that only about 10% of individuals with GTS have tics only. Factor analysis studies also indicate that tics, in particular simple motor and vocal tics, may be only one core factor of GTS (Alsobrook & Pauls 2002, Mathews et al. 2007, Robertson & Cavanna 2007, Grados & Mathews 2008, Robertson et al. 2008). This is relevant to the search for the cause of GTS. In addition, recognition of the comorbidities can have substantial influence on the management of GTS patients, and a thorough assessment of GTS patients for the presence of comorbidities is mandatory. The following will address the most important comorbidities of GTS. However, other developmental problems, e.g. dyslexia, can also coexist with GTS.

ATTENTION-DEFICIT–HYPERACTIVITY DISORDER

Attention-deficit–hyperactivity disorder represents one of the most prevalent (between 3% and 17%; Goldman et al. 1998, Barbaresi et al. 2002) and most controversial psychiatric disorders of children. Other terms that have been used to describe this disorder include attention-deficit disorder (ADD), hyperkinetic disorder (in the ICD-10 nomenclature), minimal brain dysfunction or minimal brain damage, or disorder of attention, motor control and perception (DAMP) (Landgren et al. 1996). The criteria set out in DSM-IV are the most widely used to diagnose ADHD with its key symptoms of inattention, hyperactivity and impulsivity (American Psychiatric Association 2000). For a diagnosis of ADHD, clinicians have to rely on the clinical evaluation of the child, but also on information provided by multiple informants including parents and teachers who do not always agree (Boyle et al. 1996). This is an important caveat when using the DSM-IV diagnostic algorithm.

Attention-deficit–hyperactivity disorder characteristically begins in children younger than 7 years, most commonly when children begin to walk; parents may note that children are clumsy, excessively active, impulsive with low frustration tolerance, reckless and prone to accidents. Children with ADHD may have intellectual disabilities, which at least to a degree may stem from poor concentration and the inability to finish tasks. Some form of antisocial behaviour can often be observed as the child grows up, with covert aggression, such as disobedience, cheating, lying or stealing, but also overt aggression including temper tantrums and physical aggression towards others (Hinshaw 1987, Pliszka et al. 1999, Scahill et al. 1999). The severity of the aggression-related behaviours determines whether the diagnosis of comorbid conduct disorder (CD) applies. Persistent truanting, delinquency, vandalism and destructiveness, physical aggression, bullying and spitefulness, but also sexual promiscuity among teenage girls may be apparent both at home and outside the home. According to the DSM-IV criteria, at least three out of a list of 15 such symptoms have to be present for at least 6 months; in addition, a subtype of CD, oppositional defiant disorder (ODD), can be differentiated to describe negativistic, hostile and defiant behaviour without physical aggression.

These socially unacceptable, disinhibited and sometimes aggressive behaviours often mean that, as a consequence, the child can be unpopular and thus have very few or no friends. In addition, drug and alcohol abuse are common. The prognosis depends on the severity of ADHD and comorbid CD. Adult antisocial behaviour and antisocial personality disorder may develop in almost half of children with CD (Robins 1978, Zoccolillo et al. 1992). Criminal behaviour and convictions, substance abuse and pervasive social dysfunction seem to be more common in adults who had childhood ADHD and CD (Fombonne et al. 2001a, 2001b, Stevenson & Goodman 2001). Thus childhood ADHD and CD have to be considered risk factors for adult mental health.

The comorbidity of ADHD and tic disorders is well recognised (Robertson 2006a). Between 35% and 90% of patients with GTS may also have a diagnosis of ADHD (Spencer et al. 2001), and a greater number of children with ADHD seem to develop tics compared with controls (Munir et al. 1987, Comings & Comings 1990). However, while there is no doubt that GTS, or tics, and ADHD frequently co-occur, their aetiological relationship remains unclear. ADHD symptoms tend to manifest earlier than tics and often warrant treatment with stimulants. However, there is no evidence to suggest that treatment with stimulants places children at risk of developing tics (Spencer et al. 1999, 2001). Hence the co-occurrence of ADHD and GTS or tics cannot simply be explained by the exposure to stimulants.

Attention-deficit–hyperactivity disorder is an important comorbidity to recognise in GTS. Children who suffer from the symptoms of ADHD often not only underperform academically, with subsequent disadvantages regarding their own professional development as adults, but may also be disruptive to their families and peers. Overt and covert aggression and delinquency are commonly associated with ADHD (Hinshaw 1987, Pliszka et al. 1999, Scahill et al. 1999). In GTS, ADHD, but not tics, seems to determine levels of aggressive behaviours and delinquency to a degree that is similar to children with ADHD in the absence of tics (Spencer et al. 1998, Stephens & Sandor 1999, Carter et al. 2000, Sukhodolsky et al. 2003, Rizzo et al. 2007). Children with these behaviours seem more likely to exhibit antisocial behaviours as adults (Robins 1978, Zoccolillo et al. 1992); thus the suggestion that personality disorders are more frequent in patients with GTS may in fact be due to comorbid ADHD (Robertson et al. 1997).

Like GTS, ADHD often persists into adulthood (Kessler et al. 2006). Consequently, in patients with GTS and ADHD, functional impairment and its repercussions on social interactions with peers and other family members appear to be caused by comorbid ADHD rather than tics (Dykens et al. 1990, Carter et al. 2000, Spencer et al. 2001, Haddad et al. 2009) and extend into adulthood. The majority of evidence suggests that GTS and ADHD are not genetically related (Pauls et al. 1986a). Imaging analyses suggest morphological differences between GTS and ADHD (for review see Plessen et al. 2007), whereas electrophysiologically, abnormalities in GTS+ADHD may be more widespread than in pure GTS (Orth & Rothwell 2009). Clearly, more work is needed to learn whether GTS and ADHD are two sides of the same coin or related but separate entities (Rothenberger et al. 2007).

OBSESSIVE-COMPULSIVE DISORDER

Obsessive-compulsive disorder is a common disorder affecting 2–3% of the population (American Psychiatric Association 1994). Compulsions are defined as repetitive, seemingly purposeful behaviours, which are performed according to certain rules or in a stereotyped fashion. If the ritualistic act is not executed, or is interfered with, a feeling that something terrible is about to happen may arise. This can generate extreme anxiety and uneasiness or the feeling that something is missing, all of which tend to reinforce the compulsion. Alternatively, rituals may seek to satisfy nagging doubts (e.g. reassuring oneself that the doors are locked) or patients may be extremely thorough or slow. Other rituals may be driven by obsessions, which are recurrent, intrusive and senseless thoughts. For example, excessive hand washing may result from an obsession with contamination. Obsessions and compulsions often cause a significant amount of distress to the patient, are time consuming and interfere with day-to-day functioning. In this case, a diagnosis of OCD can be made according to the criteria set out in DSM-IV (American Psychiatric Association 1994).

The cause of OCD remains unknown. Family studies suggest that OCD is a heterogeneous disorder with familial and non-familial variants (Pauls et al. 1995). Thus, at least in

TABLE 3.1
Symptom dimensions of obsessions and compulsions, and GTS

Dimension	Phenomenology	GTS
Factor I	Aggressive, sexual and religious obsessions; checking compulsions	Common
Factor II	Symmetry and ordering obsessions/compulsions	Common
Factor III	Contamination obsessions, washing/cleaning compulsions	Not common
Factor IV	Hoarding obsessions/compulsions	Not common

a subset of patients, a genetic contribution to the pathogenesis of OCD is likely. A clearer differentiation of OCD phenotypes could help the quest to identify the gene(s) that are important in this disorder. Four symptom dimensions have been identified in OCD by factorial analysis (Baer 1994, Leckman et al. 1997) (Table 3.1).

These dimensions seem to be valid over time, as suggested in a longitudinal study (Mataix-Cols et al. 2002), but have also been supported by functional imaging (Mataix-Cols et al. 2004) and treatment studies (Mataix-Cols et al. 1999). Interestingly, during development, the transient ritualistic behaviour of normal children may also follow this pattern (Evans et al. 1997, Zohar & Felz 2001).

Obsessions and compulsions are common comorbidities in patients with tics and tic disorders, including GTS. Between 25% and 50% of patients with GTS frequently reveal obsessive-compulsive behaviours (OCB) or OCD (Pauls et al. 1986b, 1991, Robertson 2000). It is not clear precisely how tic disorders and OCD are related; however, current data suggest a bidirectional association of tics and OCD with the possibility of the two disorders sharing common putative susceptibility genes (Pauls et al. 1986b).

Obsessions and compulsions, and the subjective experiences preceding compulsive repetitive behaviours, differ between patients with OCD alone and patients who have OCD and GTS, or obsessions and compulsions and GTS. In GTS, aggressive, sexual and religious obsessions and checking compulsions, and obsessions and compulsions around symmetry and ordering (including 'evening up') seem to predominate whereas contamination obsessions and washing, hoarding and collecting compulsions are more common in OCD without GTS (for a review see Robertson 2000, Table 3.2). In OCD alone, compulsions seem to be driven more often by obsessions and are more commonly associated with autonomous anxiety than in OCD with tics or GTS (Miguel et al. 1995). GTS patients often describe uncomfortable sensory phenomena, which need to be relieved by the repetitive behaviour. These sensory phenomena can be physical sensations in particular body parts, an inner mental urge or tension or a sense of being incomplete that needs to be relieved by a repetitive action (Leckman et al. 1993, Miguel et al. 1995, 2000). In addition, GTS patients often describe the need for an arrangement or a sound in an idiosyncratic way to be 'just right' (Leckman et al. 1994). This can lead to time-consuming repetitive behaviours until the look, the feel or a sound gives the 'just right' feeling. These

TABLE 3.2

Pharmacological treatment of GTS and associated conditions. The list of medications includes the drugs with which we have personal experience

Symptom	Drug	Substance class
Tics	Sulpiride	Dopamine receptor antagonist
	Haloperidol	Dopamine receptor antagonist
	Pimozide	Dopamine receptor antagonist
	Risperidone	Dopamine receptor antagonist
	Quetiapine	Dopamine receptor antagonist
	Aripiprazole	D_2-dopamine receptor antagonist, partial agonist at dopamine D_2 and serotonin 5HT-1A receptors; antagonist at serotonin 5HT-2A receptors
	Tetrabenazine	Dopamine depleting
	Clonidine	α_2-receptor agonist
	Guanfacine	α_2-receptor agonist
	Pergolide	Dopamine agonist
OCD/depression	Fluoxetine	SSRI
	Paroxetine	SSRI
	Sertraline	SSRI
	Citalopram	SSRI
	Clomipramine	Tricyclic antidepressant: Serotonin and noradrenaline reuptake inhibitor, α_1-adrenoreceptor antagonist
	Venlafaxine	Serotonin and noradrenaline reuptake inhibitor
ADHD	Methylphenidate	Stimulant
	Dexamphetamine	Stimulant
	Atomoxetine	Selective noradrenaline reuptake inhibitor
Rage/aggression	Stimulants/risperidone	

SSR, selective serotonin reuptake inhibitors.

differences between the dimensions of OCD in tic-related and non-tic related disorders could point towards factors, genetic or environmental, that differ between GTS and OCD (Leckman et al. 2003).

The sensory phenomena described by GTS patients with OCD resemble those that precede the tics. Tics and compulsions are both repetitive behaviours driven by sensory phenomena. Clinically, at times it can therefore be difficult to differentiate complex tics from compulsions.

RAGE ATTACKS

Explosive outbursts (also referred to as 'rage' or 'anger' attacks) can be observed in a substantial proportion (possibly as high as a third) of patients with TS (Bruun & Budman 1998, Budman et al. 1998, 2000). Characteristically, temper outbursts are either unprovoked or out of proportion to a minor provocation and can be associated with verbal abuse and aggressive behaviour towards objects but also other individuals (often those closest to the patient). Following the attack, the patient often is apologetic and remorseful. In GTS, an association with ADHD, OCD and particularly ODD can often be identified (Budman et al. 1998, 2000, 2003).

SELF-INJURIOUS BEHAVIOURS

Self-injurious behaviours (SIBs) describe the deliberate, non-accidental infliction of self-harm or ingestion of an overdose of a substance. The motives driving these behaviours may sometimes be difficult to identify. However, in many cases the intention of SIBs is not to commit suicide. They may signal a wish to die or be used as a means to attract attention, to escape or to manipulate others in a dysfunctional way. SIBs are non-specific and can occur in many neuropsychiatric disorders. They are particularly prevalent in mood disorders, borderline personality disorder, eating disorders and in individuals who abuse psychoactive substances. SIBs also occur in individuals with intellectual disability and organic brain disorders such as the Lesch–Nyhan syndrome, or may be driven by auditory hallucinations in schizophrenia. Apart from the defect of hypoxanthine-guanine phosphoribosyl transferase in Lesch–Nyhan syndrome that leads to excessive production of urate, the biological basis of SIBs remains unknown.

There is no classification system for SIBs. Even though four major classes of SIB – stereotypical, major, compulsive and impulsive – have been proposed, these classes overlap considerably (Favazza & Simeon 1995). The prevalence of psychiatric disorders is high in patients with SIBs (Morgan et al. 1975, Suominen et al. 1996). In addition, the risk for repetition is high and the suicide risk in a large study was found to be 2% over the 2-year study period (Isacsson et al. 1995) and may be higher over longer time periods. Thus, in a patient with SIBs a thorough evaluation of underlying psychiatric disorders is mandatory in order to provide the best possible treatment.

Gilles de la Tourette described SIBs in his original patients (Gilles de la Tourette 1885). Several subsequent studies revealed that SIBs are common in GTS (Moldofsky et al. 1974, van Woert et al. 1976, Nee et al. 1980, Stefl 1984, Robertson et al. 1997). In GTS, the character of SIBs resembles that encountered in other patient populations, possibly with the exception of drug overdoses. Patients report head banging, they hit themselves including the head and face, stab or cut themselves using sharp objects, burn themselves, e.g. with cigarettes, and a number of patients inflict injuries to their eyes (Robertson et al. 1989). These SIBs often seem to respond to an internal urge and relieve an inner tension; this is similar to the sensations that precede complex tics or compulsive behaviours. It is thus not surprising that a relationship of SIB with OCD has been reported (Robertson et al. 1989, Mathews et al. 2004). However, when distinguishing SIBs according to severity (e.g. scratching, picking at scabs or hitting versus cutting or eye poking), a close association of less severe SIBs with obsessions and compulsions was observed while the more severe SIBs correlated more with impaired impulse control (Mathews et al. 2004). However, in GTS SIBs also do occur in the context of an underlying mood disorder, in particular depression; they may be associated with the presence of substance abuse and ADHD or personality disorders.

Hence, the relationship of SIB to other psychiatric disorders needs to be clearly established in a given patient since this may have implications for management.

MOOD DISORDERS

Depression

Depression is common, with a lifetime risk of 7.5–10%, and rates are even higher in women (Kessler et al. 1997). It is also common in children, with prevalence estimates varying between 1.8% and 8.9% (Angold & Costello 1995). Depression may be mild or severe, when the lifetime suicide risk is about 15%. Depression constitutes a spectrum disorder including 'endogenous' major depressive disorder (MDD), dysthymia, residual depression, masked depression, subthreshold depression, double depression, unipolar/bipolar depression and neurotic/psychotic depression (for review see Katona & Robertson 2000, Robertson 2003). MDD may not be a disease but a syndrome, which is clinically homogeneous but aetiologically heterogeneous (Winokur 1997).

There is now good evidence from controlled and uncontrolled studies to support the view that MDD, depressive illness and depressive symptomatology are common in GTS patients (for an extensive review see Robertson & Orth 2004). In another review, depressive illness or symptomatology was shown to occur in between 13% and 76% of GTS patients and in almost all of 13 controlled studies, GTS patients had more depressive symptoms than matched controls (Robertson 2006b).

The correlates of the depression in GTS patients are increased tic severity, OCB/OCD, SIB, copro- and echophenomena, premonitory urges, sleep disturbances, the presence of conduct disorder as a youngster, aggression as well as older age and ADHD in some but not all studies (Robertson 2006b).

Depression in GTS is highly likely to be multifactorial in origin, as is the depression in non-GTS populations. Since depression is common and GTS may also be more common than was previously recognised (e.g. Mason et al. 1998, Kadesjo & Gillberg 2000, Kurlan et al. 2001, Lanzi et al. 2004), the two disorders could also coexist by chance in some instances.

Gilles de la Tourette syndrome can be a chronic, socially disabling and stigmatising disease, consequently leading to reactive depression. Many children with GTS report that they have been bullied, teased and given pejorative nicknames such as 'Noddy' or 'Nudge, nudge, wink, wink', which may have an effect on self-esteem and mood similar to other bullied children (e.g. Salmon et al. 1998, Bond et al. 2001).

The high levels of depression observed in some GTS studies (reviewed in Robertson & Orth 2004, Robertson 2006b) may have reflected the fact that patients attending specialist clinics (including GTS patients) often have more than one problem/disorder, thus introducing ascertainment bias. This view would be supported by epidemiological studies, in which individuals with GTS were not rated as having depressed mood when compared to patients without GTS or controls, and by a study in which the patients with 'pure' GTS (without comorbidity) were not more depressed than the controls (Sukhodolsky et al. 2003). OCD and ADHD, the most common comorbidities in GTS, may play a part in the aetiology of depression in GTS. Depression is the most common complication of OCD (Perugi et al. 1999, 2002, Katona & Robertson 2000), and depression is also common in ADHD (Biederman et al. 1991, Milberger et al. 1995).

The depression in patients with GTS may also be due to the side effects of medications. Depressed mood has been reported with, for example, haloperidol (Caine & Polinsky 1979, Bruun 1982), pimozide (Regeur et al. 1986, Bruggeman et al. 2001), fluphenazine (Bruun 1988), tiapride (Chouza et al. 1982), sulpiride (Robertson et al. 1990) and risperidone (Bruggeman et al. 2001, Margolese et al. 2002), and increased irritability or mood changes are a fairly common side effect of tetrabenazine (Jankovic et al. 1984).

Taken together, depressive symptoms and even MDD seem to be common in GTS. In contrast, there is no evidence to suggest that the reverse is true, i.e. GTS is more common in patients with a main diagnosis of MDD (Eapen et al. 2001). The aetiology of depression in GTS is very probably multifactorial, similar to primary depressive illness, and less likely to be caused by a single aetiological factor. A detailed assessment of depressed GTS patients can be the key to identifying and addressing factors of particular relevance to the aetiology of their depression and thus improve its recognition but also treatment and outcome.

Bipolar affective disorder
A number of case reports documented the association of bipolar affective disorder and GTS (for a review see Robertson & Orth 2004). In controlled studies the prevalence of bipolar affective disorder in patients with GTS was estimated to be around 15% (Comings & Comings 1987, Kerbeshian et al. 1995). Considering that the lifetime prevalence of bipolar affective disorder may be around 1%, this indicates that GTS and bipolar affective disorder do not co-occur by chance. Importantly, some of the comorbidities of GTS can be associated with bipolar affective disorder, in particular ADHD (e.g. Biederman et al. 1991, Hazell et al. 1999, Faraone et al. 2003, Tramontina et al. 2003, Wilens et al. 2003), conduct disorder (e.g. Kutcher et al. 1989, Kovacs & Pollock 1995, Lewinsohn et al. 1995, Biederman et al. 2003) and OCD (Chen & Dilsaver 1995, Freeman et al. 2002, Perugi et al. 2002). How GTS and bipolar affective disorder relate to each other, and whether both could be phenotypes of the same underlying putative gene(s), is not entirely clear. Nonetheless, clinicians managing patients with GTS need to be vigilant for bipolar affective disorder as a possible comorbidity in GTS (for an extensive review of this topic, see Robertson & Orth 2004).

AUTISTIC SPECTRUM DISORDERS
We do encounter patients with both GTS or tics and abnormal social development and communication difficulties. A number of these patients have difficulties engaging in warm emotional relationships and seem to be 'loners'. These characteristics are reminiscent of those encountered in autistic spectrum disorders such as childhood autism or Asperger syndrome. Indeed, there is evidence to suggest that GTS or tics may be more frequent in patients with an autistic spectrum disorder (Baron-Cohen et al. 1999a, 1999b, Canitano & Vivanti 2007). How GTS and autistic spectrum disorders relate to each other and whether they are part of the same spectrum of developmental disorders remains unclear. Nonetheless, the recognition of autistic features in a patient with GTS or the reverse may have implications for management. It is important, however, to differentiate tics from stereotypies (e.g.

hand clapping, hand waving or rocking), which are also commonly observed in autistic spectrum disorders or Rett syndrome.

Relationship between Gilles de la Tourette syndrome and its comorbidities

There is no doubt that GTS is often complicated by associated disorders such as ADHD, OCD or mood disorders. As has been discussed in each section of this chapter, the aetiological relationship of these disorders remains unclear. All these disorders are common, including GTS, so that any combination of disorders could be explained to some extent as chance co-occurrence. However, their co-occurrence is so frequent that they probably share aetiologically relevant factors.

Even though the gene(s) underlying GTS have not been identified, GTS clearly has to be viewed as an at least partly hereditary disorder with good evidence from twin and family studies supporting this view; this is true also for OCD and probably ADHD, and OCD, anxiety and depression probably share a common genetic background. Common genetic factors have been implicated as underlying the co-occurrence of tics and OCD (Pauls et al. 1986b) but have so far not been found to account for the co-occurrence of tics and ADHD. However, until the gene or genes underlying these disorders are identified, we cannot be certain whether the various disorders that make up the GTS spectrum are related to a single gene or involve multiple gene effects.

Research into the genetic basis of GTS has so far not been able to identify a single gene; several candidate genes have emerged even though no clear abnormalities have been revealed in any of the candidate genes investigated. Thus several genes may be involved in a way that has yet to be unravelled. It will be interesting to see if these genes are relevant to brain development since GTS, ADHD and OCD can be regarded as so-called developmental disorders. It is possible that the expression of these genes in relation to a particular part of the brain and/or a neuronal circuit determines the extent to which one or several of the GTS spectrum disorders occur. Interestingly, there is a striking overlap of neurobehavioural difficulties between fragile X syndrome and GTS. Fragile X syndrome is caused by a trinucleotide repeat (CGG) expansion in the first exon of the fragile X mental retardation 1 gene (*FMR1*) with subsequent loss of function of the protein product, fragile X mental retardation protein (FMRP), a protein relevant to neuronal development (Bassell & Warren 2008). Fragile X syndrome is often characterised by behaviour reminiscent of several neuropsychiatric developmental disorders including OCD, ADHD and autistic spectrum disorder, and tics can also occur in fragile X syndrome (Cornish et al. 2008, Schneider et al. 2008).

Environmental factors have also been implicated in the pathogenesis of GTS. These could include perinatal factors, such as a low birthweight with ischaemic lesions in brain parenchyma, or reduced APGAR scores 5 minutes after birth, which may predispose to the development of tics later in life (Whitaker et al. 1997, Burd et al. 1999). In addition, immunological factors have been suggested, at least in a subset of patients. To date, no clear causal relationship between these factors and tics has been established, and to our mind it would be premature to give any treatment recommendations. However, immunological factors could be a further pathogenetic player to which a genetic predisposition may have rendered individuals more vulnerable (Swedo et al. 1997, Rizzo et al 2006). Interestingly, the autoantibodies described in association with a streptococcal infection may be directed specifically at the basal ganglia. The basal ganglia are not only important within motor circuits, even though the motor cortex is their main outflow tract; they also form part of fronto-thalamo-basal ganglia-cortical circuits and have thus other functions related to mood and behaviour (Graybiel & Canales 2001, Leckman 2002). It may therefore be important in relation to the complexities of GTS spectrum disorders to discover where within these circuits a potential environmental factor exerts its effect.

Attention-deficit–hyperactivity disorder serves as a further good example to illustrate the complex relationship between genetics and the environment. While genetic factors seem to be important in ADHD, a child growing up with parents who suffer from ADHD may be subjected to significant adverse environmental influence on the acquisition of social and communication skills, with subsequent disadvantages to their mental health. The same may be true for mood disorders, in particular depression where genetic factors and the environment may have to come together. Hence, environmental factors clearly are an important component of the aetiological puzzle of GTS spectrum disorders.

Taken together, it currently remains unclear whether GTS and its associated disorders are each independent disorders that can co-occur so that one could call them true comorbidities. It is unlikely that either of the developmental syndromic entities, e.g. GTS, ADHD, OCD and others, is caused by a single-gene effect. Polygenetic effects in conjunction with, for example, environmental factors could explain the variable association of these syndromes in a multiple hit paradigm where genetic factors render individuals more susceptible to secondary factors. The individual set of symptoms, or syndromes, may point to particular brain regions or neuronal circuits that are affected during their development. A better understanding of the process of neuronal development and its regulation in different brain regions/neuronal circuits may eventually reveal whether we are looking at individual pathologies that manifest, for example, as GTS, ADHD or OCD or whether we will understand GTS spectrum disorders, or at least some of them, as a syndrome with one single underlying pathology. In the meantime, the assessment of patients has to take the individual circumstances, both genetic and environmental, of a given patient into account in order to provide the best possible care.

Management

In order to advise patients regarding the best possible treatment options, a careful and systematic clinical assessment is mandatory. It is often helpful to rank the patient's difficulties according to their own subjective impairment. It may not be easy to identify the right treatment immediately and in some patients, owing to idiosyncratic responses to medication, only a trial and error approach eventually identifies a successful choice. The decision to treat with medication must be governed by careful risk/benefit assessments with the patient, and complementary non-pharmacological treatment options, e.g. cognitive-behaviour therapy, have to be considered. In addition, particularly children with GTS and other comorbid developmental disorders may benefit greatly from a statement of special educational needs, and educating teachers and others at school can help provide a more understanding environment in which the child with GTS can thrive. Simple measures such as giving extra help and extra time in exams, a seat in front of the classroom or the option to request a time-out can be beneficial. In this chapter we will give an overview of the available treatment options for the sometimes complex symptoms and behaviours of patients with GTS. For a more detailed discussion of the treatment of GTS, we would refer the reader to a comprehensive review by one of the authors (Robertson & Stern 2000).

Aside from specific treatment of tics, general advice regarding the possible effects of stimulants other than those used for the treatment of ADHD on tic severity can be useful. Caffeine can enhance tics and is present in numerous dietary sources in addition to coffee and tea, and other recreational drugs such as speed or cocaine are potent tic-inducing agents. In contrast, maintaining an active lifestyle with ample physical activity can be beneficial for tics.

The decision to use medication for treatment needs to be considered carefully. Medications cannot cure tics, may only have moderate effects on tic severity and carry the potential to cause side effects. The pharmacological treatment of tics relies on dopamine receptor blockers such as sulpiride or haloperidol, α_2-adrenoceptor blockers, e.g. clonidine, or tetra-benazine, a dopamine-depleting drug (Table 3.2). Experience with the novel anti-psychotic drug aripiprazole suggests it may be a very useful addition to the treatment options for tics. The drug of first choice needs to take the age of the patient and the comorbidities into account. In children, and in particular those with comorbid ADHD, clonidine may be the first-line treatment. On the other hand, adolescents with both tics and troublesome rage attacks or oppositional defiant behaviour may benefit from low doses of risperidone. Other treatment options include botulinum toxin injections. In expert hands, these injections carry a low risk for side effects and they may be very useful, e.g. for loud vocalisations and coprolalia or for particularly troublesome simple motor tics such as head shaking (Cordivari et al. 2004, Porta et al. 2004). Dopamine agonists such as pergolide (Gilbert et al. 2000) can be tried if other drugs fail, and non-pharmacological treatments such as habit reversal techniques can also be useful in individual patients (Wilhelm et al. 2003). In the future, deep brain stimulation may be an alternative treatment for severely affected and otherwise treatment-refractory patients. Carefully designed trials are needed to inform us about patient selection, stimulation site and stimulation parameters (Mink et al. 2006).

Attention-deficit–hyperactivity disorder in GTS should be treated similarly to ADHD alone. Stimulants such as methylphenidate (either short release or controlled release) or dexamphetamines are the pharmacological mainstays of treatment. Recently, a non-stimulant new drug, atomoxetine, has been licensed for the treatment of ADHD in the UK, including adults. This may offer a valuable alternative in patients who do not benefit from stimulants or have unacceptable side effects. As discussed above, there is no evidence to suggest that treatment with stimulants will precipitate tics in a previously tic-free child (Spencer et al. 1999, Tourette Syndrome Study Group 2002). In addition, while in an individual patient tics may worsen following the initiation of stimulant treatment, a double-blind placebo-controlled study found no difference of the effect on tics comparing stimulant treatment and placebo (Tourette Syndrome Study Group 2002). Hence we regard the treatment of ADHD with stimulants as safe in patients with GTS. Pharmacological treatment of ADHD should be viewed as complementary to behavioural measures at school and at home that make allowances for the child's difficulties, offering extra help when needed but also a clear structure and if necessary social skills training.

Treatment of OCD in GTS does not differ from that of OCD alone. Cognitive-behaviour therapy can be very valuable and as pharmacological treatment, selective serotonin reuptake inhibitors (SSRIs) such as fluoxetine, paroxetine, sertraline and citalopram or the tricyclic clomipramine can be useful. The treatment of a mood disorder in GTS is similar to that of mood disorders without GTS.

Rage attacks and aggressive behaviours can be particularly troublesome. These behaviours have to be viewed in context with other behavioural abnormalities, in particular ADHD and CD/ODD with which they are often associated (Sukhodolsky et al. 2003). In GTS they seem often to be the result of a mixture of impaired impulse control and oppositional defiant behaviour. Treatment can aim to address the impulsivity of ADHD using stimulants but the addition of an atypical neuroleptic such as risperidone in low doses may be needed. If a combination of a stimulant and atypical neuroleptic has to be chosen, this may have the added benefit that the side effects of these medications (e.g. changes in appetite) can counteract each other. SSRIs offer an alternative. Anger management as a behavioural measure can complement pharmacological treatment, particularly in those patients who are able to identify situational triggers of their aggression.

Self-injurious behaviours can be difficult to manage. It is paramount to identify what causes these behaviours. Management and prognosis differ if, for example, SIBs occur in the context of intermittent depressive episodes, as part of compulsive or tic behaviour, impaired impulse control, or when the patient has a personality disorder or abuses psychoactive substances. If possible, pharmacological and behavioural interventions need to aim at the underlying causes. However, there are patients in whom SIBs prove difficult to control, in particular in those patients who are at risk of inflicting severe self-injuries, e.g. when they suffer the urge to injure their eyes, protective glasses or splints that prevent the fingers from reaching the eyes may have to be used.

The treatment of children with psychotropic medication can at times be unavoidable. However, most drugs have to be prescribed off label because they are not licensed for use in children. Little is known about the long-term effects of these drugs when given to the developing brain. However, in our experience the use of these medications is not any less safe than in adults provided that children are monitored carefully. Nonetheless, considerable controversies have arisen following the reporting of aggressive behaviours and suicide of children treated with SSRIs for depression (for a detailed discussion see, for example, Check 2004, Klein 2004). It is not yet entirely clear whether a causal relationship between medication and aggression or suicide can be established. SSRIs have been very valuable in the treatment of depression and OCD and their safety profile, in particular regarding overdoses, offers advantages over other antidepressants, e.g. tricyclic antidepressants. Thus we continue to use SSRIs in our young patients in particular for the treatment of OCD; however, extra caution with dosages and close monitoring of children who commence treatment with SSRIs are mandatory, especially when treating depression.

REFERENCES

Alsobrook JP 2nd, Pauls DL (2002) A factor analysis of tic symptoms in Gilles de la Tourette's syndrome. *Am J Psychiatr* **159**, 291–296.

American Psychiatric Association (1994) *Diagnostic and Statistical Manual of Mental Disorders*, 4th edn. Washington, DC: American Psychiatric Association.

American Psychiatric Association (2000) *Diagnostic and Statistical Manual of Mental Disorders*, 4th edn, revised. Washington, DC: American Psychiatric Association.

Angold A, Costello EJ (1995) Developmental epidemiology. *Epidemiol Rev* **17**, 74–82.

Baer L (1994) Factor analysis of symptom subtypes of obsessive compulsive disorder and their relation to personality and tic disorders. *J Clin Psychiatr* **55**(suppl), 18–23.

Barbaresi WJ, Katusic SK, Colligan RC, et al. (2002) How common is attention-deficit/hyperactivity disorder? Incidence in a population-based birth cohort in Rochester, Minn. *Arch Pediatr Adolesc Med* **156**, 217–224.

Baron-Cohen S, Mortimore C, Moriarty J, Izaguirre J, Robertson M (1999a) The prevalence of Gilles de la Tourette's syndrome in children and adolescents with autism. *J Child Psychol Psychiatr* **40**, 213–218.

Baron-Cohen S, Scahill VL, Izaguirre J, Hornsey H, Robertson MM (1999b) The prevalence of Gilles de la Tourette syndrome in children and adolescents with autism: a large scale study. *Psychol Med* **29**, 1151–1159.

Bassell GJ, Warren ST (2008) Fragile X syndrome: loss of local mRNA regulation alters synaptic development and function. *Neuron* **60**, 201–214.

Biederman J, Newcorn J, Sprich S (1991) Comorbidity of attention deficit hyperactivity disorder with conduct, depressive, anxiety, and other disorders. *Am J Psychiatr* **148**, 564–577.

Biederman J, Mick E, Wozniak J, Monuteaux MC, Galdo M, Faraone SV (2003) Can a subtype of conduct disorder linked to bipolar disorder be identified? Integration of findings from the Massachusetts General Hospital Pediatric Psychopharmacology Research Program. *Biol Psychiatr* **53**, 952–960.

Bliss J (1980) Sensory experiences of Gilles de la Tourette syndrome. *Arch Gen Psychiatr* **37**, 1343–1347.

Bond L, Carlin JB, Thomas L, Rubin K, Patton G (2001) Does bullying cause emotional problems? A prospective study of young teenagers. *BMJ* **323**, 480–484.

Boyle MH, Offord DR, Racine Y, Szatmari P, Fleming JE, Sanford M (1996) Identifying thresholds for classifying childhood psychiatric disorder: issues and prospects. *J Am Acad Child Adolesc Psychiatr* **35**, 1440–1448.

Bruggeman R, van der Linden C, Buitelaar JK, Gericke GS, Hawkridge SM, Temlett JA (2001) Risperidone versus pimozide in Tourette's disorder: a comparative double-blind parallel-group study. *J Clin Psychiatr* **62**, 50–56.

Bruun RD (1982) Dysphoric phenomena associated with haloperidol treatment of Tourette syndrome. *Adv Neurol* **35**, 433–436.

Bruun RD (1988) Subtle and underrecognized side effects of neuroleptic treatment in children with Tourette's disorder. *Am J Psychiatr* **145**, 621–624.

Bruun RD, Budman CL (1998) Paroxetine treatment of episodic rages associated with Tourette's disorder. *J Clin Psychiatr* **59**, 581–584.

Budman CL, Bruun RD, Park KS, Olson ME (1998) Rage attacks in children and adolescents with Tourette's disorder: a pilot study. *J Clin Psychiatr* **59**, 576–580.

Budman CL, Bruun RD, Park KS, Lesser M, Olson M (2000) Explosive outbursts in children with Tourette's disorder. *J Am Acad Child Adolesc Psychiatr* **39**, 1270–1276.

Budman CL, Rockmore L, Stokes J, Sossin M (2003) Clinical phenomenology of episodic rage in children with Tourette syndrome. *J Psychosom Res* **55**, 59–65.

Burd L, Severud R, Klug MG, Kerbeshian J (1999) Prenatal and perinatal risk factors for Tourette disorder. *J Perinat Med* **27**, 295–302.

Caine ED, Polinsky RJ (1979) Haloperidol-induced dysphoria in patients with Tourette syndrome. *Am J Psychiatr* **136**, 1216–1217.

Canitano R, Vivanti G (2007) Tics and Tourette syndrome in autism spectrum disorders. *Autism* **11**(1), 19–28.

Carter AS, O'Donnell DA, Schultz RT, Scahill L, Leckman JF, Pauls DL (2000) Social and emotional adjustment in children affected with Gilles de la Tourette's syndrome: associations with ADHD and family functioning. *J Child Psychol Psychiatr* **41**, 215–223.

Check E (2004) Antidepressants: bitter pills. *Nature* **431**, 122–124.

Chen YW, Dilsaver SC (1995) Comorbidity for obsessive-compulsive disorder in bipolar and unipolar disorders. *Psychiatr Res* **59**, 57–64.

Chouza C, Romero S, Lorenzo J, et al. (1982) [Clinical trial of tiapride in patients with dyskinesia (author's transl)]. *Sem Hop* **58**, 725–733.

Comings BG, Comings DE (1987) A controlled study of Tourette syndrome. V. Depression and mania. *Am J Hum Genet* **41**, 804–821.

Comings DE, Comings BG (1990) A controlled family history study of Tourette's syndrome, I: Attention-deficit hyperactivity disorder and learning disorders. *J Clin Psychiatr* **51**, 275–280.

Cordivari C, Misra VP, Catania S, Lees AJ (2004) New therapeutic indications for botulinum toxins. *Mov Disord* **19**, S157–161.

Cornish K, Turk J, Hagerman R (2008) The fragile X continuum: new advances and perspectives. *J Intellect Disabil Res* **52**, 469–482.

Dykens E, Leckman J, Riddle M, Hardin M, Schwartz S, Cohen D (1990) Intellectual, academic, and adaptive functioning of Tourette syndrome children with and without attention deficit disorder. *J Abnorm Child Psychol* **18**, 607–615.

Eapen V, Laker M, Anfield A, Dobbs J, Robertson MM (2001) Prevalence of tics and Tourette syndrome in an inpatient adult psychiatry setting. *J Psychiatr Neurosci* **26**, 417–420.

Evans DW, Leckman JF, Carter A, et al. (1997) Ritual, habit, and perfectionism: the prevalence and development of compulsive-like behavior in normal young children. *Child Dev* **68**, 58–68.

Faraone SV, Glatt SJ, Tsuang MT (2003) The genetics of pediatric-onset bipolar disorder. *Biol Psychiatr* **53**, 970–977.

Favazza AR, Simeon D (1995) Self-mutilation. In: Hollander E, Stein DJ (eds) *Impulsivity and Aggression*. Chichester: John Wiley, pp.185–200.

Fombonne E, Wostear G, Cooper V, Harrington R, Rutter M (2001a) The Maudsley long-term follow-up of child and adolescent depression. 1. Psychiatric outcomes in adulthood. *Br J Psychiatr* **179**, 210–217.

Fombonne E, Wostear G, Cooper V, Harrington R, Rutter M (2001b) The Maudsley long-term follow-up of child and adolescent depression. 2. Suicidality, criminality and social dysfunction in adulthood. *Br J Psychiatr* **179**, 218–223.

Freeman MP, Freeman SA, McElroy SL (2002) The comorbidity of bipolar and anxiety disorders: prevalence, psychobiology, and treatment issues. *J Affect Disord* **68**, 1–23.

Freeman RD, Fast DK, Burd L, Kerbeshian J, Robertson MM, Sandor P (2000) An international perspective on Tourette syndrome: selected findings from 3,500 individuals in 22 countries. *Dev Med Child Neurol* **42**, 436–447.

Gilbert DL, Sethuraman G, Sine L, Peters S, Sallee FR (2000) Tourette's syndrome improvement with pergolide in a randomized, double-blind, crossover trial. *Neurology* **54**, 1310–1315.

Gilles de la Tourette G (1885) Etude sur une affection nerveuse caracterisee par de l'incoordination motrice accompagnee d'echolalie et de coprolalie. *Arch Neurol (Paris)* **9**, 19–42, 158–200.

Goldman LS, Genel M, Bezman RJ, Slanetz PJ (1998) Diagnosis and treatment of attention-deficit/ hyperactivity disorder in children and adolescents. Council on Scientific Affairs, American Medical Association. *JAMA* **279**, 1100–1107.

Grados MA, Mathews CA (2008) Latent class analysis of Gilles de la Tourette syndrome using comorbidities: clinical and genetic implications. *Biol Psychiatr* **64**, 219–225.

Graybiel AM, Canales JJ (2001) The neurobiology of repetitive behaviors: clues to the neurobiology of Tourette syndrome. *Adv Neurol* **85**, 123–131.

Haddad ADM, Umoh G, Bhatia V, Robertson MM (2009) Adults with Tourette's syndrome with and without attention deficit hyperactivity disorder. *Acta Psychiatr Scand* **120**(4), 299–307.

Hazell PL, Lewin TJ, Carr VJ (1999) Confirmation that Child Behavior Checklist clinical scales discriminate juvenile mania from attention deficit hyperactivity disorder. *J Paediatr Child Health* **35**, 199–203.

Hinshaw SP (1987) On the distinction between attentional deficits/hyperactivity and conduct problems/ aggression in child psychopathology. *Psychol Bull* **101**, 443–463.

Isacsson G, Wassermann D, Bergman U (1995) Self-poisoning with antidepressants and other psychotropics in an urban area of Sweden. *Ann Clin Psychiatr* **7**, 113–118.

Jankovic J (1997) Tourette syndrome. Phenomenology and classification of tics. *Neurol Clin* **15**, 267–275.

Jankovic J (2001) Differential diagnosis and etiology of tics. *Adv Neurol* **85**, 15–29.

Jankovic J, Glaze DG, Frost JD Jr (1984) Effect of tetrabenazine on tics and sleep of Gilles de la Tourette's syndrome. *Neurology* **34**, 688–692.

Kadesjo B, Gillberg C (2000) Tourette's disorder: epidemiology and comorbidity in primary school children. *J Am Acad Child Adolesc Psychiatr* **39**, 548–555.

Katona C, Robertson MM (2000) *Psychiatry at a Glance*. London: Blackwell Science.

Kerbeshian J, Burd L, Klug MG (1995) Comorbid Tourette's disorder and bipolar disorder: an etiologic perspective. *Am J Psychiatr* **152**, 1646–1651.

Kessler RC, Zhao S, Blazer DG, Swartz M (1997) Prevalence, correlates, and course of minor depression and major depression in the National Comorbidity Survey. *J Affect Disord* **45**, 19–30.

Kessler RC, Adler L, Barkley R, et al. (2006) The prevalence and correlates of adult ADHD in the United States: results from the National Comorbidity Survey Replication. *Am J Psychiatr* **163**, 716–723.

Khalifa N, von Knorring AL (2005) Tourette syndrome and other tic disorders in a total population of children: clinical assessment and background. *Acta Paediatr* **94**, 1608–1614.

Klein DF (2004) SSRIs in children and suicide. *Science* **305**, 1401.

Kovacs M, Pollock M (1995) Bipolar disorder and comorbid conduct disorder in childhood and adolescence. *J Am Acad Child Adolesc Psychiatr* **34**, 715–723.

Kurlan R, Daragjati C, Como PG, et al. (1996) Non-obscene complex socially inappropriate behavior in Tourette's syndrome. *J Neuropsychiatr Clin Neurosci* **8**, 311–317.

Kurlan R, McDermott MP, Deeley C, et al. (2001) Prevalence of tics in schoolchildren and association with placement in special education. *Neurology* **57**, 1383–1388.

Kutcher SP, Marton P, Korenblum M (1989) Relationship between psychiatric illness and conduct disorder in adolescents. *Can J Psychiatr* **34**, 526–529.

Landgren M, Pettersson R, Kjellman B, Gillberg C (1996) ADHD, DAMP and other neurodevelopmental/psychiatric disorders in 6-year- old children: epidemiology and comorbidity. *Dev Med Child Neurol* **38**, 891–906.

Lanzi G, Zambrino CA, Termine C, et al. (2004) Prevalence of tic disorders among primary school students in the city of Pavia, Italy. *Arch Dis Child* **89**, 45–47.

Leckman JF (2002) Tourette's syndrome. Lancet **360**, 1577–1586.

Leckman JF, Walker DE, Cohen DJ (1993) Premonitory urges in Tourette's syndrome. *Am J Psychiatr* **150**, 98–102.

Leckman JF, Walker DE, Goodman WK, Pauls DL, Cohen DJ (1994) 'Just right' perceptions associated with compulsive behavior in Tourette's syndrome. *Am J Psychiatr* **151**, 675–680.

Leckman JF, Grice DE, Boardman J, et al. Symptoms of obsessive-compulsive disorder. *Am J Psychiatr* **154**, 911–917.

Leckman JF, Zhang H, Vitale A, et al. (1998) Course of tic severity in Tourette syndrome: the first two decades. *Pediatrics* **102**, 14–19.

Leckman JF, Peterson BS, King RA, Scahill L, Cohen DJ (2001) Phenomenology of tics and natural history of tic disorders. *Adv Neurol* **85**, 1–14.

Leckman JF, Pauls DL, Zhang H, et al. (2003) Obsessive-compulsive symptom dimensions in affected sibling pairs diagnosed with Gilles de la Tourette syndrome. *Am J Med Genet* **116**, 60–68.

Lewinsohn PM, Klein DN, Seeley JR (1995) Bipolar disorders in a community sample of older adolescents: prevalence, phenomenology, comorbidity, and course. *J Am Acad Child Adolesc Psychiatr* **34**, 454–463.

Margolese HC, Annable L, Dion Y (2002) Depression and dysphoria in adult and adolescent patients with Tourette's disorder treated with risperidone. *J Clin Psychiatr* **63**, 1040–1044.

Mason A, Banerjee S, Eapen V, Zeitlin H, Robertson MM (1998) The prevalence of Tourette syndrome in a mainstream school population. *Dev Med Child Neurol* **40**, 292–296.

Mataix-Cols D, Rauch SL, Manzo PA, Jenike MA, Baer L (1999) Use of factor-analyzed symptom dimensions to predict outcome with serotonin reuptake inhibitors and placebo in the treatment of obsessive-compulsive disorder. *Am J Psychiatr* **156**, 1409–1416.

Mataix-Cols D, Rauch SL, Baer L, et al. (2002) Symptom stability in adult obsessive-compulsive disorder: data from a naturalistic two-year follow-up study. *Am J Psychiatr* **159**, 263–268.

Mataix-Cols D, Wooderson S, Lawrence N, Brammer MJ, Speckens A, Phillips ML (2004) Distinct neural correlates of washing, checking and hoarding symptom dimensions in obsessive-compulsive disorder. *Arch Gen Psychiatr* **61**, 564–576.

Mathews CA, Waller J, Glidden D, et al. (2004) Self injurious behaviour in Tourette syndrome: correlates with impulsivity and impulse control. *J Neurol Neurosurg Psychiatr* **75**, 1149–1155.

Mathews CA, Jang KL, Herrera LD, et al. (2007) Tic symptom profiles in subjects with Tourette syndrome from two genetically isolated populations. *Biol Psychiatr* **61**, 292–300.

Miguel EC, Coffey BJ, Baer L, Savage CR, Rauch SL, Jenike MA (1995) Phenomenology of intentional repetitive behaviors in obsessive- compulsive disorder and Tourette's disorder. *J Clin Psychiatr* **56**, 246–255.

Miguel EC, do Rosario-Campos MC, Prado HS, et al. (2000) Sensory phenomena in obsessive-compulsive disorder and Tourette's disorder. *J Clin Psychiatr* **61**, 150–156; quiz 157.

Milberger S, Biederman J, Faraone SV, Murphy J, Tsuang MT (1995) Attention deficit hyperactivity disorder and comorbid disorders: issues of overlapping symptoms. *Am J Psychiatr* **152**, 1793–1799.

Mink JW, Walkup J, Frey KA, et al. Patient selection and assessment recommendations for deep brain stimulation in Tourette syndrome. *Mov Disord* **21**(11), 1831–1838.

Moldofsky H, Tullis C, Lamon R (1974) Multiple tic syndrome (Gilles de la Tourette's syndrome). *J Nerv Ment Disord* **159**, 282–292.

Morgan HG, Burns-Cox CJ, Pocock H, Pottle S (1975) Deliberate self-harm: clinical and socio-economic characteristics of 368 patients. *Br J Psychiatr* **127**, 564–574.

Munir K, Biederman J, Knee D (1987) Psychiatric comorbidity in patients with attention deficit disorder: a controlled study. *J Am Acad Child Adolesc Psychiatr* **26**, 844–848.

Nee LE, Caine ED, Polinsky RJ, Eldridge R, Ebert MH (1980) Gilles de la Tourette syndrome: clinical and family study of 50 cases. *Ann Neurol* **7**, 41–49.

Orth M, Rothwell JC (2009) Motor cortex excitability and comorbidity in Gilles de la Tourette syndrome. *J Neurol Neurosurg Psychiatr* **80**, 29–34.

Pappert EJ, Goetz CG, Louis ED, Blasucci L, Leurgans S (2003) Objective assessments of longitudinal outcome in Gilles de la Tourette's syndrome. *Neurology* **61**, 936–940.

Pauls DL, Hurst CR, Kruger SD, Leckman JF, Kidd KK, Cohen DJ (1986a) Gilles de la Tourette's syndrome and attention deficit disorder with hyperactivity. Evidence against a genetic relationship. *Arch Gen Psychiatr* **43**, 1177–1179.

Pauls DL, Towbin KE, Leckman JF, Zahner GE, Cohen DJ (1986b) Gilles de la Tourette's syndrome and obsessive-compulsive disorder. Evidence supporting a genetic relationship. *Arch Gen Psychiatr* **43**, 1180–1182.

Pauls DL, Raymond CL, Stevenson JM, Leckman JF (1991) A family study of Gilles de la Tourette syndrome. *Am J Hum Genet* **48**, 154–163.

Pauls DL, Alsobrook JP 2nd, Goodman W, Rasmussen S, Leckman JF (1995) A family study of obsessive-compulsive disorder. *Am J Psychiatr* **152**, 76–84.

Perugi G, Akiskal HS, Ramacciotti S, et al. (1999) Depressive comorbidity of panic, social phobic, and obsessive-compulsive disorders re-examined: is there a bipolar II connection? *J Psychiatr Res* **33**, 53–61.

Perugi G, Toni C, Frare F, Traverso MC, Hantouche E, Akiskal HS (2002) Obsessive-compulsive-bipolar comorbidity: a systematic exploration of clinical features and treatment outcome. *J Clin Psychiatr* **63**, 1129–1134.

Peterson BS, Leckman JF (1998) The temporal dynamics of tics in Gilles de la Tourette syndrome. *Biol Psychiatr* **44**, 1337–1348.

Plessen KJ, Royal JM, Peterson BS (2007) Neuroimaging of tic disorders with co-existing attention-deficit/ hyperactivity disorder. *Eur Child Adolesc Psychiatr* **16**, 60–70.

Pliszka SR, Carlson CL, Swanson JM (1999) *ADHD with Comorbid Disorders: Clinical Assessment and Management.* New York: Guilford.

Porta M, Maggioni G, Ottaviani F, Schindler A (2004) Treatment of phonic tics in patients with Tourette's syndrome using botulinum toxin type A. *Neurol Sci* **24**, 420–423.

Regeur L, Pakkenberg B, Fog R, Pakkenberg H (1986) Clinical features and long-term treatment with pimozide in 65 patients with Gilles de la Tourette's syndrome. *J Neurol Neurosurg Psychiatr* **49**, 791–795.

Rizzo R, Gulisano M, Pavone P, Fogliani F, Robertson MM (2006) Increased antistreptoccal antibody titres and anti-basal ganglia antibodies in Tourette's syndrome: a controlled study. *J Child Neurol* **21**(9), 747–753.

Rizzo R, Curatolo P, Gulisano M, Virzi M, Arpino C, Robertson MM (2007) Disentangling the effects of Tourette syndrome and attention deficit hyperactivity disorder on cognitive and behavioral phenotypes. *Brain Dev* **29**, 413–420.

Robertson MM. Annotation: Gilles de la Tourette syndrome – an update. *J Child Psychol Psychiatr* **35**, 597–611.

Robertson MM (2000) Tourette syndrome, associated conditions and the complexities of treatment. *Brain* **123**(Pt 3), 425–462.

Robertson MM (2003) Diagnosing Tourette syndrome: is it a common disorder? *J Psychosom Res* **55**, 3–6.

Robertson MM (2006a) Attention deficit hyperactivity disorder, tics and Tourette's syndrome: the relationship and treatment implications. A commentary. *Eur Child Adolesc Psychiatr* **15**, 1–11.

Robertson MM (2006b) Mood disorders and Gilles de la Tourette's syndrome: an update on prevalence, etiology, comorbidity, clinical associations, and implications. *J Psychosom Res* **61**, 349–358.

Robertson MM, Cavanna AE (2007) The Gilles de la Tourette syndrome: a principal component factor analytic study of a large pedigree. *Psychiatr Genet* **17**, 143–152.

Robertson MM, Orth M (2006) Behavioural and affective disorders in Tourette syndrome. In: Walkup JT, Mink JW, Hollenbeck PJ, editors. Tourette Syndrome. Advances in Neurology 2006. Philadephia: Lippincott Williams & Wilkins.

Robertson MM, Stern JS (2000) Gilles de la Tourette syndrome: symptomatic treatment based on evidence. *Eur Child Adolesc Psychiatr* **9**, I60–75.

Robertson MM, Trimble MR, Lees AJ (1989) Self-injurious behaviour and the Gilles de la Tourette syndrome: a clinical study and review of the literature. *Psychol Med* **19**, 611–625.

Robertson MM, Schnieden V, Lees AJ (1990) Management of Gilles de la Tourette syndrome using sulpiride. *Clin Neuropharmacol* **13**, 229–235.

Robertson MM, Banerjee S, Hiley PJ, Tannock C (1997) Personality disorder and psychopathology in Tourette's syndrome: a controlled study. *Br J Psychiatr* **171**, 283–286.

Robertson MM, Althoff RR, Hafez A, Pauls DL (2008) Principal components analysis of a large cohort with Tourette syndrome. *Br J Psychiatr* **193**, 31–36.

Robins LN (1978) Sturdy childhood predictors of adult antisocial behaviour: replications from longitudinal studies. *Psychol Med* **8**, 611–622.

Rothenberger A, Roessner V, Banaschewski T, Leckman J (2007) Co-existence of tic disorders and attention-deficit/hyperactivity disorder-recent advances in understanding and treatment. *Eur Child Adolesc Psychiatr* **16**, I/1-I/4.

Salmon G, James A, Smith DM (1998) Bullying in schools: self reported anxiety, depression, and self esteem in secondary school children. BMJ **317**, 924–925.

Scahill L, Schwab-Stone M, Merikangas KR, Leckman JF, Zhang H, Kasl S (1999) Psychosocial and clinical correlates of ADHD in a community sample of school-age children. *J Am Acad Child Adolesc Psychiatr* **38**. 976–984.

Schneider SA, Robertson MM, Rizzo R, Turk J, Bhatia KP, Orth M (2008) Fragile X syndrome associated with tic disorders. *Mov Disord* **23**, 1108–1112.

Spencer T, Biederman J, Harding M, et al. (1998) Disentangling the overlap between Tourette's disorder and ADHD. *J Child Psychol Psychiatr* **39**, 1037–1044.

Spencer T, Biederman M, Coffey B, Geller D, Wilens T, Faraone S (1999) The 4-year course of tic disorders in boys with attention-deficit/hyperactivity disorder. *Arch Gen Psychiatr* **56**, 842–847.

Spencer T, Biederman J, Coffey B, Geller D, Faraone S, Wilens T (2001) Tourette disorder and ADHD. *Adv Neurol* **85**, 57–77.

Stefl ME (1984) Mental health needs associated with Tourette syndrome. *Am J Public Health* **74**, 1310–1313.

Stephens RJ, Sandor P (1999) Aggressive behaviour in children with Tourette syndrome and comorbid attention-deficit hyperactivity disorder and obsessive-compulsive disorder. *Can J Psychiatr* **44**, 1036–1042.

Stevenson J, Goodman R (2001) Association between behaviour at age 3 years and adult criminality. *Br J Psychiatr* **179**, 197–202.

Sukhodolsky DG, Scahill L, Zhang H, et al. (2003) Disruptive behavior in children with Tourette's syndrome: association with ADHD comorbidity, tic severity, and functional impairment. *J Am Acad Child Adolesc Psychiatr* **42**: 98–105.

Suominen K, Henriksson M, Suokas J, Isometsa E, Ostamo A, Lonnqvist J (1996) Mental disorders and comorbidity in attempted suicide. *Acta Psychiatr Scand* **94**, 234–240.

Swedo SE, Leonard HL, Mittleman BB, et al. (1997) Identification of children with pediatric autoimmune neuropsychiatric disorders associated with streptococcal infections by a marker associated with rheumatic fever. *Am J Psychiatr* **154**, 110–112.

Tourette Syndrome Study Group (2002) Treatment of ADHD in children with tics: a randomized controlled trial. *Neurology* **58**, 527–536.

Tramontina S, Schmitz M, Polanczyk G, Rohde LA (2003) Juvenile bipolar disorder in Brazil: clinical and treatment findings. *Biol Psychiatr* **53**, 1043–1049.

Van Woert MH, Jutkowitz R, Rosenbaum D, Bowers MB Jr (1976) Gilles de la Tourette's syndrome: biochemical approaches. *Res Publ Assoc Res Nerv Ment Dis* **55**, 459–465.

Whitaker AH, van Rossem R, Feldman JF, et al. (1997) Psychiatric outcomes in low-birth-weight children at age 6 years: relation to neonatal cranial ultrasound abnormalities. *Arch Gen Psychiatr* **54**, 847–856.

Wilens TE, Biederman J, Wozniak J, Gunawardene S, Wong J, Monuteaux M (2003) Can adults with attention-deficit/hyperactivity disorder be distinguished from those with comorbid bipolar disorder? Findings from a sample of clinically referred adults. *Biol Psychiatr* **54**, 1–8.

Wilhelm S, Deckersbach T, Coffey BJ, Bohne A, Peterson AL, Baer L (2003) Habit reversal versus supportive psychotherapy for Tourette's disorder: a randomized controlled trial. *Am J Psychiatr* **160**, 1175–1177.

Winokur G (1997) All roads lead to depression: clinically homogeneous, etiologically heterogeneous. *J Affect Disord* **45**, 97–108.

Zoccolillo M, Pickles A, Quinton D, Rutter M (1992) The outcome of childhood conduct disorder: implications for defining adult personality disorder and conduct disorder. *Psychol Med* **22**, 971–986.

Zohar AH, Felz L (2001) Ritualistic behavior in young children. *J Abnorm Child Psychol* **29**, 121–128.

4
COMORBIDITY IN NEURODEVELOPMENTAL DISORDERS: THE CASE OF ATTENTION-DEFICIT– HYPERACTIVITY DISORDER

Eric Taylor

Most children with the symptoms of attention-deficit–hyperactivity disorder (ADHD) show signs of other diagnoses as well. This has been the conclusion of several reviews – see, for instance, Gillberg et al. (2004) – and it is the starting point for this one.

The frequency of associated problems has given rise to uncertainty and confusion in the treatment of ADHD. Complex cases may not have the ADHD component recognised or may have it treated in ways that miss the other conditions. Families can be confused if the children receive multiple labels, especially when they seem contradictory.

Some of the confusion arises simply from the word 'comorbidity'. This implies that separate disorders are present – and this begs the question of whether the disorders are in truth separate. It may be, for instance, that an apparently separate disorder (such as emotional disturbance) is actually a part of the ADHD complex, subject to the same rules and the same interventions, and that its separation into a distinct condition is an artefact of clumsy classification schemes.

True 'comorbidity' only really arises when it is already plain that there is a validated distinction between ADHD and the other condition. More broadly, we can distinguish several reasons why people with ADHD might also meet criteria for another diagnosis. There are several mechanisms, the key ones being as follows.

- Invalid distinctions between diagnoses.
- Referral and other selection bias.
- Criterion overlap, i.e. the same clinical features are taken as evidence for more than one diagnosis. One diagnosis is a complication of the other.
- One diagnosis gives rise to a 'phenocopy' of the other, i.e. a superficially similar set of problems but with different underlying pathology.
- There are risk factors in common.
- There is a separate third condition that gives rise to features of both.

In different circumstances all these possibilities can apply. Rhee (2005) has reviewed some of them and emphasised that they can be difficult to tell apart.

Impact of classification schemes on comorbidity

The taxonomy of child mental health has had to base itself almost entirely on descriptions of behaviour. Aetiological classifications were attempted early in the development of the profession (along the lines of 'minimal brain dysfunction' or 'developmental fixation') but proved too unreliable to sustain a useful discourse. The answer to the problem of disagreement between clinicians was a return to the simpler level of patterns of behaviour. This is not a total picture – a few diagnoses such as 'reactive attachment disorder' or 'post-traumatic stress disorder' do include a presumed aetiology – but it applies to the conditions being described here. It is not intended to be a permanent arrangement – a good classification will be based on pathophysiological disturbance – but it is necessary for the moment.

One result of a descriptive classification is that there is no conceptual difficulty about combining a descriptive psychiatric diagnosis such as ADHD with an aetiological, neurological one such as fragile X. They are incommensurable descriptions and both need recognising. If only one can be chosen, there will be disagreement on which to choose so the preferred taxonomy is multiaxial and both can be coded.

Another result of descriptive classification is that different patterns of symptoms can be described that are in fact manifestations of the same condition. In the past, for example, a good deal of distinction was made between 'hyperactive' and 'hyper-reactive' types of disturbance. The distinction was never shown to predict a different course or aetiology and indeed, most children with clear and pervasive hyperactivity proved also to be unduly reactive to the environment. The distinction is therefore not made in classification any more. In thinking about other overlaps with ADHD, we shall have to consider whether the other condition is indeed a separate condition or just part of an ADHD complex.

Classification schemes also allow the possibility of criterion overlap. Ordinarily, some effort is made to ensure that the same behaviours do not enter into the criteria for more than one disorder, because it is evident that confusion will result. Sometimes, however, overlap creeps in. The criteria for bipolar disorder were developed for adult classification, while the criteria for ADHD came from child specialists. As will be seen below, the same behaviours came to be taken as features of both.

The nature of classification schemes therefore carries some responsibility for unwanted and misleading overlaps between psychiatric categories. They cannot, however, take all the blame. Mental problems do very frequently coexist, and clinical practice must reckon with them.

Three kinds of ADHD association – with other neurodevelopmental problems, with other psychiatric disorders and with illnesses of the brain – require separate consideration.

Associations with other neurodevelopmental problems

The different neurodevelopmental disorders have many features in common. All, by definition, are of early onset with tendencies for disability to continue. All are very much more common in boys than in girls. (The exception, Rett syndrome, is only encountered in girls; the x-linked mutation is lethal in males.) All are associated with each other. All show substantial genetic influences; it is not yet clear how far those genetic differences are specific to the individual disorders.

One therefore needs to ask, first, whether the disorders should all be seen as one vulnerability. Usually they should not. There are clear distinctions, in brain anatomy, neurochemistry and response to medication. Second, are they independent? In other words, is each of the two components of a mixed presentation similar to its non-comorbid form? Third, why do they associate together?

PERVASIVE DEVELOPMENTAL DISORDERS

Attention-deficit–hyperactivity disorder can validly be distinguished from autism, so the association between the disorders does not stem merely from making false distinctions within a broad group of severe developmental problems.

The evidence comes from several sources. At the level of brain structure, people with ADHD have in general shown reduced volumes – especially in right frontal brain regions, caudate, corpus callosum and cerebellum but also in parietal, temporal and occipital brain regions (Castellanos et al. 2002, Sowell et al. 2003). The largest structural study conducted so far using combined cross-sectional and longitudinal design revealed that these volumetric abnormalities seem to be evident early in life, persist with age, and show parallel and non-progressive developmental growth curves (except for the caudate where group differences disappeared with age) (Castellanos et al. 2002). In autism, by contrast, anatomical studies have found *larger* total brain and white matter volumes in most cortical brain regions and in the cerebellum, caudate and globus pallidum (Piven et al. 1996). One shared anatomical dysmorphology between autism and ADHD appears to be a smaller corpus callosum (Saitoh et al. 1995) but this is commonly a rather non-specific concomitant of problems elsewhere in the brain.

At the neuropsychological level, executive function deficits are common in autism as well as in ADHD (Pennington & Ozonoff 1996). Children with autism also show problems that are much less associated with ADHD – in theory of mind and in weak central coherence (Booth et al. 2003). A few studies have compared autism and ADHD directly, but results are somewhat contradictory. Ozonoff & Jensen (1999) found a double dissociation between both disorders: children with autism showed difficulties in planning and cognitive flexibility but not in inhibition, whereas children with ADHD showed the opposite pattern. On the other hand, Nyden et al. (1999) failed to replicate this finding: in their study both ADHD and autism were associated with a response inhibition deficit and only children with ADHD showed deficits in flexibility. Geurts et al. (2004) also failed to obtain a double dissociation: children with autism demonstrated deficits in all executive function (EF) domains, except interference control and working memory; ADHD was associated with EF deficits in inhibiting a prepotent response and verbal fluency.

At a genetic level, cosegregation of ADHD and autism has not been demonstrated. Nevertheless, several regions of the chromosomes which have been suggested to harbour risk genes for autism – 2q24, 15q, 6p13, 17p11 – have also been highlighted in genome-wide scans for ADHD (Smalley et al. 2002). These investigations are at an early stage and it may turn out that commonality of genes simply reflects an imprecision in the characterisation of cases, rather than the operation of non-specific genetic risk factors.

Comparison of the comorbid group with the 'pure' groups has not yet yielded clear conclusions on whether they simply show the coexistence of two separate problems. In the important matter of treatment response, the autistic component and the ADHD component often vary independently. Clinically, it can be valuable to treat the ADHD component when it is there: stimulants can give a good response. Some special considerations, however, apply. Stimulants can also provoke an increase in social withdrawal and stereotyped behaviour – as is to be expected from their dopaminergic actions. Drugs with less dopaminergic activity, such as atomoxetine and imipramine, might seem more logical, but trial evidence is lacking and clinical experience suggests they are often disappointing. Sedative drugs have a place when the child's overactivity is agitated in quality, and sometimes when stimulants and atomoxetine fail. Risperidone is probably the most often used and perhaps the most effective but clonidine is a safer alternative and is often worth trying first.

There is, however, an important qualifier to make to this general conclusion of two different conditions linked by correlated causes. Not all overactive children in the autism spectrum are the same. There are other patterns as well as the disorganised, impulsive, context-dependent qualities that characterise ADHD. Some children with autism show a driven, unvarying pattern of incessant activity, often rather stereotyped in form. This has not received formal investigation, but clinicians will recognise it as a problem of a rather different kind, and one that is often refractory to stimulant medication. Other children in the autism spectrum present with episodic overactivity, sometimes undirected and extreme in degree, sometimes ended by a seizure. Catatonic overactivity is then a possible diagnosis (with bipolar disorder in the differential) and a trial of lorazepam will sometimes be helpful and support the diagnosis.

SPECIFIC LEARNING DISABILITIES (SLD)
The structural brain changes described in reading disabilities (RD) are rather different from those mentioned above for ADHD: they include reduced volume in the brain regions that mediate speech and learning, such as the bilateral inferior prefrontal lobes (pars triangularis), anterior lobe of the cerebellum, and left hemispheric temporal and parietal brain regions (Pennington et al. 1999, Klingberg et al. 2000, Pernet et al. 2009).

At the neuropsychological level, there are differences as well as similarities. The clearest distinction probably comes from the problems that are more specific to RD: deficits in phonological processing (Wagner & Torgesen 1987, Pennington et al. 1993), auditory temporal processing (Tallal 1980), rapid sequential processing (Wagner & Torgesen 1987) and the automatisation of skills (Nicolson et al. 2001). Individuals with RD are also impaired in several abilities in which children with ADHD are also weak: processing speed (Tannock et al. 2000, Rucklidge & Tannock 2002), time processing (Smith et al. 2002), verbal working memory (Rucklidge & Tannock 2002, Willcutt et al. 2002a), cognitive flexibility (Weyandt et al., 1998), planning (Klorman et al. 1999), and response inhibition (Purvis & Tannock 2000, Willcutt et al. 2002a). The research, however, has not always been rigorous in excluding minor degrees of inattentiveness and impulsiveness from the RD group, and the tests used are not always comparable – the time-processing deficit in RD may affect much shorter intervals (tens of milliseconds) than the difficulty in discriminating intervals in the hundreds-of-milliseconds range that characterises ADHD.

If we can regard them as distinct entities, why are they so often associated? Genetically, there may be some influences in common. A quantitative trait locus study revealed significant linkage of a chromosome 6p region to both disorders (Willcutt et al. 2002b). More recently, suggestive linkage to RD was found in four chromosomal regions, including regions on 16p and 17q that had previously been implicated in ADHD (Loo et al. 2004).

Another possible reason for the association is the phenocopy hypothesis: that in the comorbid state, the inattentiveness of behaviour at school is a consequence of the difficulty of concentrating when material is presented verbally. In other words, the inattentive behaviour may be secondary to the reading disorder rather than similar to other forms of ADHD. This possibility seemed to get strong support from a study by Pennington et al. (1993), who reported that the comorbid group exhibited significant phonological processing deficits (like RD) but *not* the EF deficits typically associated with ADHD. This finding has not, however, been replicated and it may have been an artefact of subject selection (the children were in remedial education groups). Most later studies with larger samples found that the comorbid group exhibited the deficits of both single groups in an additive fashion (Rucklidge & Tannock 2002, Willcutt et al. 2002a).

Nevertheless, inattentive behaviour may be secondary to specific intellectual disabilities in some defined situations, especially for the subgroup of inattentive children whose problems only appear in school. Both clinical and epidemiological studies have suggested that hyperactivity confined to the school situation is more likely than other presentations of hyperactivity to have an onset after the age of school entry and an association with reading problems (Taylor et al. 1986, Ho et al. 1996). It is tempting to suppose that in this case the hyperactive behaviour is secondary to academic failure.

For some subgroups of children, reading problems may be worsened by ADHD. Remedial teachers and language therapists are often frustrated in their attempts to teach by the inattentiveness of the child. Conversely, inattentiveness is only to be expected if the material to be learned is pitched at too high a level for the child to manage. But, in general, clinicians should not try to explain away one problem as being the result of the other. Chadwick et al. (1999) followed a community sample of children with hyperactive behaviour over a 10-year period. The outcome, by comparison with ordinary children from similar backgrounds, suggested that reading problems and hyperactive behaviour pursued independent courses after the age of 7, without an interactive effect from the coexistence of both problems.

In clinical practice, both difficulties should be recognised. In particular, the presence of SLD should not be a barrier to giving medication for ADHD. In a predictive study, reading problems did not predict drug actions one way or the other (Taylor et al, 1987). This again emphasises the frequent independence of the two problems, and the value of recognising and treating both.

TOURETTE DISORDER

Hyperactive behaviour is a common association of Tourette disorder (TD). Robertson (2006) provides a full review. The picture is diagnostically complicated, because hyperactivity may be the initial presentation in a child whose TD will appear only later (and sometimes be misinterpreted as an adverse reaction to stimulants). It is quite possible to overlook TD in the initial presentation of hyperkinetic disorder. The tics are often not very salient and the pathognomonic features, such as vocal tics, may not yet have appeared.

The contrasts between ADHD and TD have not received enough research attention for a full review to be useful, and what neurobiological research exists is somewhat contradictory. The developmental courses are different: the fluctuations in TD are not paralleled by ADHD. Clinically they seem like very different presentations, but one source of confusion needs to be guarded against: multiple and minor tics may be misinterpreted as the restlessness and fidgetiness of ADHD, if the repetitive quality of the tics is not appreciated. In cases of doubt, it can be valuable to videotape sequences of the child's behaviour. Review may well indicate the repetitiveness that is a hallmark of tics.

Clinical opinion, and scientific evidence, vary about the reason for the association. Family studies are conflicting about whether the linkage between the two is attributable to common genetic influences. In practice, when both problems are present together, then it is usually best to make a dual diagnosis. The two aspects of the child's disorder will need separate planning, and the sometimes adverse effect of stimulants upon tics may lead to management problems. Stimulants are not contraindicated, and some authorities have found that they are no more likely than placebo to generate tic disorders, but in the long term some individuals show compelling evidence of a relationship between stimulants and tics and the prescriber will need to consider atomoxetine or nicotine patches when the treatment target is ADHD. Sometimes prescribers make an early recourse to neuroleptics such as risperidone or sulpiride on the basis that both conditions may be ameliorated, but this can lead to unnecessary hazards of medication.

GLOBAL INTELLECTUAL DISABILITIES

The presence of generalised intellectual diability is often due to a disorder of brain development (see below). Indeed, when the IQ is below 50, there is almost always a structural brain abnormality. ADHD can therefore be another consequence of the underlying cause.

Special difficulties arise in the definition. The criteria for hyperactivity and inattention, in both ICD-10 and DSM-IV, include a requirement that the problems should be abnormal for the developmental stage of the individual. This is not an easy judgement, and even the conceptual basis is unclear. Some degree of inattentiveness is, almost by definition, to be expected in people with intellectual disability. Should one take, for example, a cut-off at the level defining the worst 5% of the population at a given level of intellectual disability? To do so would beg the question of whether ADHD is more common in intellectual disability and ignores the possibility that impaired attention might depress the IQ. Treatable problems might then go untreated.

A useful rule of thumb is to estimate the mental age of the child, and judge the presence of impairment on the basis of what would be expected from a normally intelligent child at that chronological age. There are clearly untested assumptions here. A child of 10 with a mental age of 5 years is not the same as an average child aged 5 years. It would be helpful for research to focus more on the development of normative value in representative populations. In the meantime, there is little substitute for clinical experience.

The treatment of ADHD in children with low IQ follows similar principles to those in the normally intelligent. Trial evidence is scanty but suggests that stimulants are superior to placebo. Adverse effects of drugs, however, are not well quantified and clinical experience suggests that they may be somewhat more common in those with brain abnormalities. The balance of benefit and risk may therefore tilt towards interventions other than medication but medication remains a valuable tool.

The difficulty of distinguishing hyperactive behaviour from other forms of disruptiveness is also greater than in the normally intelligent. In the absence of self-report, mania may go unrecognised. The frequent presence of autistic features can complicate the recognition of coexistent hyperactivity. Challenging behaviour without hyperactivity is not expected to be sensitive to stimulants or atomoxetine; behaviour therapy is then the most effective intervention, and clinical trials indicate that risperidone has a greater effect than placebo.

The difficulties inherent in assessment mean that a trial of medication often needs to be carried out before the diagnosis is secure. It becomes all the more important that monitoring is careful and, at least in the early stages, frequent.

Common disorders of mental health

The common problems of mental health – conduct and oppositional disorders and emotional disorders involving anxiety or depression – are also disproportionately common in children with ADHD. Indeed, oppositional behaviour is virtually the rule in referred children with ADHD, so that many clinicians find it unnecessary to code the oppositionality separately.

Many of the risk factors for the behaviour and emotional disorders of childhood are rather diffuse in their effects. Environmental stressors typically raise the risk of a wide variety of problems. This is not to say that there is no specificity at all; the risk factors for conduct disorder (harsh discipline, neglect, social adversity) are not identical to the risk factors for the emotional disorders (such as parental mental disorder). Nevertheless, the different kinds of social adversity are very frequently found together and have similar roots.

CONDUCT PROBLEMS

More evidence has accumulated about the overlap of hyperactivity and conduct disorder than any other combination of problems. The association is strong, both in boys (Taylor et al. 1991) and in girls (Young et al. 2005).

They are not, however, simply different ways of labelling the same problem. In some studies, the distinction has been blurred by reporting individuals with conduct disorder who also shared hyperactive behaviour or individuals with ADHD who were not free of conduct problems. Nevertheless, a community survey of about 3000 6–8 year olds in East London was able to identify children with pure forms of each type of problem, and compare them with age-matched controls who shared both problems and a sample of those sharing neither problem (Taylor et al. 1991). The results showed that the presence of hyperactivity, whether or not conduct problems were also present, predicted high rates of neurodevelopmental problems such as language delay and clumsiness; conduct problems without hyperactivity did not. A similar conclusion can be taken from responsiveness to methylphenidate: hyperactivity predicts responsiveness even for non-hyperactive behaviour problems. Children with conduct problems but no hyperactivity are less responsive (Taylor et al. 1987).

At a neuropsychological level, too, most studies have found that deficits in executive function are found in ADHD but not in oppositional conduct disorders without hyperactivity. With almost 400 children included, the largest study found evidence for planning deficits in children with ADHD combined type (not inattentive type) that were independent of oppositional and conduct disorders (Klorman et al. 1999). Cognitive flexibility did not discriminate between groups. Clark et al. (2000) found that adolescents with ADHD performed worse on two EF measures, independently of oppositional defiant disorder (ODD)/conduct disorder (CD). Similar results were obtained using three different measures of working memory (WM) (Kalff et al. 2002). In a meta-analysis of the Stop Task (response inhibition), Oosterlaan et al. (1998) at first concluded that both disorders are associated with inhibitory deficits but more recent studies, taking better account of the tendency for those diagnosed as ODD to have high levels of hyperactive behaviour, showed that ADHD, but not ODD or CD, was associated with inhibitory dysfunction (Oosterlaan & Sergeant 1998, Kooijmans et al. 2000, Schachar et al. 2000).

There may still be some cognitive deficits affecting those with oppositional/conduct problems but no ADHD. Aronowitz et al. (1994) found that CD was associated with poor cognitive flexibility (Wisconsin Card Sorting Test) and visuospatial problems (Rey-Osterreith Complex Figure Test). Nevertheless, the validity of the distinction between ADHD and CD seems clear. It is not always easy to make in practice: unwary diagnosticians may confuse complaints of non-compliant behaviour with the impulsive disorganisation of ADHD but it is important to make the distinction.

Genetically, however, the two problems are not well distinguished. A cross-twin cross-trait analysis carried out on a general population sample suggested, for example, that genetic influences operating on CD (at least during the period from the ages of 7 to 14) are similar to those operating on ADHD (Nadder et al. 2002).

The apparent contradiction can be resolved in one of two ways. First, the coexistence of both could be a separate type of disorder. Some investigators (e.g. Biederman et al. 1992, Faraone et al. 1998) have found a particularly high rate of affected relatives in the 'comorbid' group, and suggest it may be a subtype characterised by a higher genetic loading. The studies, however, give information about familiality rather than heritability. The antisocial relatives of the combined group might have transmitted their problems socially rather than genetically.

The second explanation for the clinical dissimilarity but genetic similarity of the two problems is that hyperactivity is a genetically influenced basis of both, and conduct problems arise as a complication – whether because of additional genetic influences or via the mediation of hostile reactions with family members and peers. In support of this is the longitudinal finding (in the East London study mentioned above) that hyperactivity predicts the later emergence of conduct problems, but not vice versa (Taylor et al, 1996).

Clinically, there is a reasonable consensus among expert guideline papers: when both hyperactivity and conduct problems are present together, then the hyperactivity should usually be treated first, with subsequent review of how much conduct problem is left and, if necessary, the addition of behaviour modification approaches – often in family format. This advice is based on guidelines for school-age children. In young children, the best performing intervention in clinical trials is 'parent training' and this targets both oppositional and hyperactive behaviour together.

EMOTIONAL PROBLEMS

About a quarter of children with diagnosed ADHD show emotional problems too. There are several distinct patterns that need to be distinguished, but often are not.

First, many children with ADHD show a pattern of emotional dyscontrol. They react unpredictably and with great intensity, but transiently, to events affecting them. The emotion is appropriate but its expression is excessive. Their tantrums are extreme and easily provoked, their fears lead to insistently avoidant behaviour; but the mood states last at most for a few hours. This pattern may well be an intrinsic part of ADHD; intuitively it seems close to the lack of inhibition that affects their rule-governed behaviour. Research has not yet clarified whether it should be seen as a separate problem. Mood-stabilising drugs are often given (e.g. valproate, risperidone) but their potential for toxicity suggests that a trial of stimulants will usually be the first line of medication.

Second, a substantial minority show enduring states of anxiety and/or depression; they resemble other children with anxiety-based disorders, and separation anxiety and (in older children) social anxiety are common. The evocation of distress is predictable and its expression is often less flamboyant than in the 'dyscontrol' group described above. In this group, the treatment will follow the principles of treatment in non-hyperactive children, with cognitive approaches to dealing with anxiety-laden situations and gradual exposure to them. In predictive trials, the presence of such high levels of anxiety predicts a poor response to stimulant medication (Taylor et al. 1987). In the influential MTA trial, children with comorbid emotional problems did better with carefully crafted medication than with intensive psychosocial treatment but they did particularly poorly if placed in the trial arm in which treatment as usual was given in the community (usually involving medication) (MTA Co-operative Group 1999).

In short, stimulants and atomoxetine are not contraindicated when comorbid anxiety is present, but they may not work, and carefully monitored and finely adjusted doses are advisable. If they do not work, then a sedative such as clonidine or an anxiolytic such as fluoxetine is usually the next choice.

A third, and more recently recognised, pattern is that of bipolar disorder. Classically (bipolar I disorder), this involves elation and grandiosity of mood and a course of distinct episodes lasting for several days at least. Less typically (bipolar not otherwise specified or bipolar NOS), the episodes are brief – and in some descriptions they may be very brief, with several episodes a day. Furthermore, the mood may not be elated but consist solely of irritability (an easy provocation to anger). This bipolar NOS is clearly very similar to the first patterns described above, of emotional dyscontrol, and with present knowledge it seems best to treat accordingly, pending the results of ongoing research to clarify whether it should be treated as bipolar I. When bipolar I is present, it should be treated as in adults with mood-stabilising drugs (lithium, anticonvulsants such as valproate or lamotrigine, risperidone).

Associations with brain disorders

Overactivity, restlessness and inattentiveness are all common associations of some brain diseases, including epilepsy, hydrocephalus, hemiplegia, developmental co-ordination disorder, phenylketonuria and mucopolysaccharidosis. One common reason is that the brain illness has affected structures that are involved in the normal control of activity and attention. This is not necessarily a specific change, and the same illnesses that give rise to ADHD may also give rise to generalised intellectual impairment (see above). Clinicians need to distinguish between the generalised effects and any specific impairment of attention; IQ testing is therefore a necessary part of the assessment.

In the case of brain injury or insult rising from environmental causes, then further complexities need to be considered. Hyperactive behaviour can be associated because it has brought about the injury rather than because it is a result. Recklessness in children can make them more prone to being knocked over by cars, falling out of trees or getting themselves exposed to lead in dust from old paint (Taylor & Warner Rogers 2005). Careful history taking is needed.

The general lesson for diagnosis is that the brain disorder is not an alternative to ADHD. ADHD is not a neurological diagnosis but a description of behaviour; it may still be present whatever neurological condition is present too, and in general its symptomatic treatment follows the same principles as would be the case in children with otherwise normal brains. It is also helpful to make an individual formulation of the developmental pathways through which the ADHD has arisen, and we now consider the possibilities for the most common associated neurological problem: epilepsy.

ADHD AND EPILEPSY

Attention-deficit–hyperactivity disorder is commonly found in children who demonstrate epilepsy. For example, Dunn et al. (2003) studied 175 children with epilepsy in the age range of 9–14 years. They found that 20 met the DSM-IV criteria for ADHD combined type, 42 for the predominantly inattentive type, and four for the hyperactive impulsive type. Sex, type of seizure and focus of discharge were not predictors of ADHD within the group with epilepsy.

It is not possible to give a rigorous view from this investigation about the extent of the risk that epilepsy imposes. The absence of a control group in that study, as in others on ADHD and epilepsy, makes it impossible to interpret clearly. Plainly, a rate of more than one-third of children showing behavioural symptomatology is strikingly high but in the absence of pathognomonic grounds for the diagnosis and a considerable range for uncertainty – as evidenced in the wide variety of prevalence rates for ADHD reported from different epidemiological surveys – it is conceivable that the same measures might have identified a comparable number in a group of children with otherwise normal brains.

Nevertheless, clinical experience is in keeping with such an observation and the neuro-psychiatric surveys carried out in the Isle of Wight two generations ago confirm that hyper-kinetic disorder (a severe form of ADHD) was not only more common in people with epilepsy but disproportionately more common, i.e. accounting for a greater proportion of diagnosis (Rutter et al. 1970).

There are several possible reasons for this and all of them may be encountered in individual cases. First, there is a group of causes that can be seen as being mediated by abnormal brain mechanisms. The genetic and environmental factors that are risk factors for epilepsy may also determine the presence of ADHD. More directly, subclinical seizures can in themselves impair concentration. Clinically this can be difficult: an absence seizure may be hard to distinguish from a micro-lapse of attention, and simultaneous behavioural and EEG recording is often necessary to make the distinction. Nevertheless, it is plain that for children with poorly controlled epilepsy, the presence of large numbers of epileptic discharges can in itself produce an impairment of attention that is improved by treatment with antiepileptic drugs. More generally, seizures can have an impact upon broader mental function. A good example would be the association of frequent spike-and-wave activity during sleep with behavioural disturbance in the daytime.

An underlying neurological disease may account for both epilepsy and ADHD. An epileptic focus, say in the frontal lobe, may be reflecting underlying structural damage that would also be capable of producing ADHD symptoms even if epilepsy were not a consequence.

A more indirect route involving brain mechanisms is that the toxic effects of anticon-vulsant drugs may in themselves produce symptoms of ADHD. Furthermore, non-compliance with medication may be a result of ADHD and therefore lead to poorer seizure control and an apparent association between severity of epilepsy and ADHD symptomatology.

All these possibilities need to be considered in the individual case before one needs to invoke a possible commonality of neurophysiological process. It is easy to speculate that an impaired ability to inhibit might underline both disinhibitory symptoms of ADHD and the failure to control the brain's discharges in epilepsy – but this would imply a very speculative identification of overall inhibitory mechanism that has no route in known neuroscience.

As well as these brain mechanisms, there are a number of extracerebral mechanisms that could account for associations between ADHD and epilepsy in individual cases. The presence of ADHD probably restricts the access to other kinds of intervention. Parents may be less able to take their children to diagnostic services or less able to achieve satisfactory compliance with medication. Reduced access to treatment may therefore mean that the association between the presence of seizures and the presence of ADHD reflects a failure adequately to control either or both.

There are other, more speculative, pathways. It may also be that ADHD entails some impairment of the ability to suppress seizures. The presence of seizures may make it more likely that ADHD is recognised – recognition might be improved because health services are involved, the tolerance of parents for disruptive behaviour might be reduced or they may be more likely to attribute behaviour to a medical cause, when epilepsy is present as well. Epilepsy may also evoke a pathogenic environment. Family relationships are not in themselves thought to create ADHD, but they can certainly modulate its impact and therefore its presentation to services, and the presence of high critical expressed emotion is a mediator of the course of children with ADHD, making it more likely that they will develop antisocial symptoms, and therefore that they will remain in touch with services.

Clinically, it should also be remembered that the apparent symptoms of ADHD may in fact be representing a different sort of symptomatology. Another neurodevelopmental disorder, associated with the brain changes of epilepsy, may be masquerading (see above).

With all these possible reasons for association, it is perhaps not surprising that research has found it difficult to make general conclusions about the reasons for the overlap. Such research progress may well depend upon the more systematic and explicit delineation of these possible routes of association. Meanwhile, from the perspective of clinical practice, the need remains for some subtlety of analysis of each individual case. The therapeutic interventions for ADHD in children with epilepsy may include increasing the anticonvulsant dosage (to achieve better control of seizures, e.g. at night-time), the reduction of anticonvulsant medication (to avoid toxicity to which high blood levels and low folate levels may be a clue), the exhibition of stimulants (which are not contraindicated in epilepsy, contrary to the teachings of many textbooks), the counselling of parents and others concerning the nature of the child's problems, or more focused measures (such as expressed emotion reduction) to modify the impact of relationship adversity upon the child, the introduction of specific behaviour therapy, and the treatment (with drugs or other methods) of the disorders such as mania that have masqueraded as ADHD in the first place.

General conclusions

The diagnosis of ADHD is not simply a matter of recognising its core features, if that were all that was needed, then it could usually be coped with satisfactorily in primary care. Good clinical assessment needs to reckon with the range of other factors that can be present, either as differential diagnosis or associated problem. A full assessment will formulate the reasons why the other problems are present: this, as much as their description, will guide treatment.

The most common reasons for the comorbidities are as follows.

- They are separate disorders with linked causes – as we have seen for other neurodevelopmental disorders. The implication is that the management of the associated disorder will need to be part of the treatment plan from the start.
- The associated disorders have arisen because ADHD is a risk factor for their development. This will apply particularly for problems such as oppositional behaviour disorders and substance misuse. The appropriate management will often be to treat the ADHD first, but to take pains to review the outcome for whether the complicating disorder has indeed improved or needs separate management in its own right.
- The pattern of ADHD symptoms is broader than recognised by the diagnostic schemes and includes, for instance, emotional volatility and dyscontrol. The key will often be

careful management of the ADHD, but with attention to monitoring the full range of problems and not merely the core behaviours included in commercial rating scales.

• ADHD can result from a wide range of brain disorders for complex reasons and a comprehensive management is required.

For all these reasons, the services provided for ADHD need to have a general competence in the recognition and treatment of associated mental and physical disorders. The training of staff, and the skill mix within a service, need to go beyond the core of ADHD symptoms and specific therapies.

REFERENCES

Aronowitz B, Liebowitz M, Hollander E, et al. (1994) Neuropsychiatric and neuropsychological findings in conduct disorder and attention-deficit hyperactivity disorder. *J Neuropsychiatr Clin Neurosci* **6**(3), 245–249.

Biederman J, Faraone SV, Keenan K, et al. (1992) Further evidence for family-genetic risk factors in attention deficit hyperactivity disorder. Patterns of comorbidity in probands and relatives psychiatrically and pediatrically referred samples. *Arch Gen Psychiatr* **49**(9), 728–738.

Booth R, Charlton R, Hughes C, Happe F (2003) Disentangling weak coherence and executive dysfunction: planning drawing in autism and attention-deficit/hyperactivity disorder. *Philos Trans R Soc Lond B Biol Sci* **358**(1430), 387–392.

Castellanos FX, Lee PP, Sharp W, et al. (2002) Developmental trajectories of brain volume abnormalities in children and adolescents with attention-deficit/hyperactivity disorder. *JAMA* **288**(14), 1740–1748.

Clark C, Prior M, Kinsella GJ (2000) Do executive function deficits differentiate between adolescents with ADHD and oppositional defiant/conduct disorder? A neuropsychological study using the Six Elements Test and Hayling Sentence Completion Test. *J Abnorm Child Psychol* **28**(5), 403–414.

Dunn DW, Austin JK, Harezlak J, Ambrosius WT (2003) ADHD and epilepsy in childhood. *Dev Med Child Neurol* 45(1), 50–54.

Faraone SV (2004) Genetics of adult attention-deficit/hyperactivity disorder. *Psychiatr Clin North Am* 27, 303–321.

Faraone SV, Biederman J, Mennin D, Russell R, Tsuang MT (1998) Familial subtypes of attention deficit hyperactivity disorder: a 4-year follow-up study of children from antisocial-ADHD families. *J Child Psychol Psychiatr* **39**(7), 1045–1053.

Geurts HM, Verte S, Oosterlaan J, Roeyers H, Sergeant JA (2004) How specific are executive functioning deficits in attention deficit hyperactivity disorder and autism? *J Child Psychol Psychiatr* **45**(4), 836–854.

Gillberg C, Gillberg IC, Rasmussen P (2004) Co-existing disorders in ADHD – implications for diagnosis and intervention. *Eur Child Adolesc Psychiatr* **13**(Suppl 1), I80–92.

Ho TP, Luk ESL, Leung PWL, Taylor E, Mak FL, Bacon-Shone J (1996) Situational versus pervasive hyperactivity in a community sample. *Psychol Med* 26, 309–321.

Kalff AC, Hendriksen JG, Kroes M, et al. (2002) Neurocognitive performance of 5- and 6-year-old children who met criteria for attention deficit/hyperactivity disorder at 18 months follow-up: results from a prospective population study. *J Abnorm Child Psychol* **30**(6), 589–598.

Klingberg T, Hedehus M, Temple E, et al. (2000) Microstructure of temporo-parietal white matter as a basis for reading ability: evidence from diffusion tensor magnetic resonance imaging. *Neuron* **25**(2), 493–500.

Klorman R, Hazel-Fernandez LA, Shaywitz SE, et al. (1999) Executive functioning deficits in attention-deficit/hyperactivity disorder are independent of oppositional defiant or reading disorder. *J Am Acad Child Adolesc Psychiatr* **38**(9), 1148–1155.

Kooijmans R, Scheres A, Oosterlaan J (2000) Response inhibition and measures of psychopathology: a dimensional analysis. *Neuropsychol Dev Cogn Sect C Child Neuropsychol* **6**(3), 175–184.

Loo SK, Fisher SE, Francks C, et al. (2004) Genome-wide scan of reading ability in affected sibling pairs with attention-deficit/hyperactivity disorder: unique and shared genetic effects. *Mol Psychiatr* **9**(5), 485–493.

MTA Cooperative Group (1999) A 14-month randomized clinical trial of treatment strategies for attention-deficit/hyperactivity disorder. Multimodal Treatment Study of Children with ADHD. *Arch Gen Psychiatr* **56**, 1073–1086.

Nadder TS, Rutter M, Silberg JL, Maes HH, Eaves LJ (2002) Genetic effects on the variation and covariation of attention deficit-hyperactivity disorder (ADHD) and oppositional-defiant disorder/conduct disorder (ODD/CD) symptomatologies across informant and occasion of measurement. *Psychol Med* **32**(1), 39–53.

Nicolson RI, Fawcett AJ, Dean P (2001) Developmental dyslexia: the cerebellar deficit hypothesis. *Trends Neurosci* **24**(9), 508–511.

Nyden A, Gillberg C, Hjelmquist E, Heiman M (1999) Executive function/attention deficits in boys with Asperger syndrome, attention disorder and reading/writing disorder. *Autism* **3**, 213–228.

Oosterlaan J, Sergeant JA (1998) Effects of reward and response cost on response inhibition in AD/HD, disruptive, anxious, and normal children. *J Abnorm Child Psychol* **26**(3), 161–174.

Oosterlaan J, Logan GD, Sergeant, JA (1998) Response inhibition in AD/HD, CD, comorbid AD/HD + CD, anxious, and control children: a meta-analysis of studies with the stop task. *J Child Psychol Psychiatr* **39**(3), 411–425.

Ozonoff S, Jensen J (1999) Brief report: specific executive function profiles in three neurodevelopmental disorders. *J Autism Dev Disord* **29**(2), 171–177.

Pennington BF, Ozonoff S (1996) Executive functions and developmental psychopathology. *J Child Psychol Psychiatr* **37**(1), 51–87.

Pennington BF, Groisser D, Welsh MC (1993) Contrasting cognitive deficits in attention deficit hyperactivity disorder versus reading disability. *Dev Psychol* **29**, 511–523.

Pennington BF, Filipek PA, Lefly D, et al. (1999) Brain morphometry in reading-disabled twins. *Neurology* **53**(4), 723–729.

Pernet CR, Poline JB, Domonet JF, Rousselet GA (2009) Brain classification reveals the right cerebellum as the best biomarker of dyslexia. *BMC Neurosci* **10**, 67.

Piven J, Arndt S, Bailey J, Andreasen N (1996) Regional brain enlargement in autism: a magnetic resonance imaging study. *J Am Acad Child Adolesc Psychiatr* **35**(4), 530–536.

Purvis KL, Tannock R (2000) Phonological processing, not inhibitory control, differentiates ADHD and reading disability. *J Am Acad Child Adolesc Psychiatr* **39**(4), 485–494.

Rhee SH, Hewitt JK, Corley RP, Willcutt EG, Pennington BF (2005) Testing hypotheses regarding the causes of comorbidity: examining the underlying deficits of comorbid disorders. *J Abnorm Psychol* **114**(3), 346–362.

Robertson MM (2006) Attention deficit hyperactivity disorder, tics and Tourette's syndrome: the relationship and treatment implications. A commentary. *Eur Child Adolesc Psychiatr* **15**(1), 1–11.

Rucklidge JJ, Tannock R (2002) Neuropsychological profiles of adolescents with ADHD: effects of reading difficulties and gender. *J Child Psychol Psychiatr* **43**(8), 988–1003.

Rutter M, Graham P, Yule W (1970) *A Neuropsychiatric Study in Childhood.* Clinics in Developmental Medicine, Nos. 35/36. London: SIMP/Heinemann.

Saitoh O, Courchesne E, Egaas B, Lincoln AJ, Schreibman L (1995) Cross-sectional area of the posterior hippocampus in autistic patients with cerebellar and corpus callosum abnormalities. *Neurology* **45**(2), 317–324.

Schachar R, Mota VL, Logan GD, Tannock R, Klim P (2000) Confirmation of an inhibitory control deficit in attention-deficit/hyperactivity disorder. *J Abnorm Child Psychol* **28**(3), 227–235.

Smalley SL, Kustanovich V, Minassian SL, et al. (2002) Genetic linkage of attention-deficit/hyperactivity disorder on chromosome 16p13, in a region implicated in autism. *Am J Hum Genet* **71**(4), 959–963.

Smith A, Taylor E, Rogers JW, Newman S, Rubia K (2002) Evidence for a pure time perception deficit in children with ADHD. *J Child Psychol Psychiatr* **43**(4), 529–542.

Sowell ER, Thompson PM, Welcome SE, Henkenius AL, Toga AW, Peterson BS (2003) Cortical abnormalities in children and adolescents with attention-deficit hyperactivity disorder. *Lancet* **362**(9397), 1699–1707.

Stevenson J, Pennington BF, Gilger JW, DeFries JC, Gillis JJ (1993) Hyperactivity and spelling disability: testing for shared genetic aetiology. *J Child Psychol Psychiatr* **34**(7), 1137–1152.

Tallal P (1980) Auditory temporal perception, phonics, and reading disabilities in children. *Brain Lang* **9**(2), 182–198.

Tannock R, Martinussen R, Frijters J (2000) Naming speed performance and stimulant effects indicate effortful, semantic processing deficits in attention-deficit/hyperactivity disorder. *J Abnorm Child Psychol* **28**(3), 237–252.

Taylor E, Warner Rogers J (2005) Practitioner review: early adversity and developmental disorders. *J Child Psychol Psychiatr Allied Disc* **46**, 451–467.

Taylor E, Everitt B, Thorley G, Schachar R, Rutter M, Wieselberg M (1986) Conduct disorder and hyperactivity: II. A cluster analytic approach to the identification of a behavioral syndrome. *Br J Psychiatr* **149**, 768–777.

Taylor E, Schachar R, Thorley G, Wieselberg HM, Everitt B, Rutter M (1987) Which boys respond to stimulant medication? A controlled trial of methylphenidate in boys with disruptive behaviour. *Psychol Med* **17**, 121–143.

Taylor E, Sandberg S, Thorley G, Giles S (1991) *The Epidemiology of Childhood Hyperactivity*. Maudsley Monograph No. 33. Oxford: Oxford University Press.

Taylor E, Chadwick O, Heptinstall E, Danckaerts M (1996) Hyperactivity and conduct problems as risk factors for adolescent development. *J Am Acad Child Adolesc Psychiatr* **35**, 1213–1226.

Wagner RK, Torgesen JK (1987) The nature of phonological processing and its causal role in the acquisition of reading skills. *Psychol Bull* **101**, 192–212.

Weyandt LL, Rice JA, Linterman I, Mitzlaff L, Emert E (1998) Neuropsychological performance of a sample of adults with ADHD, developmental reading disorder, and controls. *Dev Neuropsychol* **14**, 643–656.

Willcutt EG, Pennington BF, DeFries JC (2000) Twin study of the etiology of comorbidity between reading disability and attention-deficit/hyperactivity disorder. *Am J Med Genet* **96**(3), 293–301.

Willcutt EG, DeFries JC, Pennington BF, Olson RK, Smith SD, Cardon LR (2002a) Genetic etiology of comorbid reading difficulties and ADHD. In: Plomin R, DeFries JC, McGuffin P, Craig I (eds) *Behavioral Genetics in a Postgenomic Era*. Washington, DC: American Psychiatric Association, pp. 227–246.

Willcutt EG, Pennington BF, Smith SD, et al. (2002) Quantitative trait locus for reading disability on chromosome 6p is pleiotropic for attention-deficit/hyperactivity disorder. *Am J Med Genet* **114**(3), 260–268.

Young S, Heptinstall E, Sonuga-Barke EJS, Chadwick O, Taylor E (2005) The adolescent outcome of hyperactive girls: self-report of psychosocial status. *J Child Psychol Psychiatr Allied Disc* **46**, 255–262.

5

EARLY LANGUAGE DISORDER AS A FREQUENT COMORBIDITY IN MANY DEVELOPMENTAL DISORDERS IN YOUNG CHILDREN

Isabelle Rapin

Preliminary comment regarding comorbidity

We have created clean diagnostic 'boxes' to classify developmental disorders, for example developmental language disorder, intellectual disability, attention-deficit disorder, autism. We have operationalised the criteria for creating clear boundaries to each 'box' so that it appears to be a 'diagnosis'. This has greatly enhanced communication among professionals and fostered research on well-defined populations. Diagnostic labels play a critical role in securing medical and educational services, and for communicating with parents and professionals whose main concern is not nosologic classification. We need to keep in mind, however, that although there are many prototypical exemplars of children who fit our boxes perfectly, there are also many children who do not: some children might just as well be put into one as another box or into several boxes; others may not meet strict criteria for any box and remain in diagnostic limbo, with the consequence that their needs may not be met.

It is to children who might fit two or more boxes that we assign several comorbid labels. Some of these children do have dual or multiple independent diagnoses, like the proverbial measles and broken leg; in others one brain disorder, for example a genetically caused brain anomaly or a congenital or early brain lesion, may cause what seem to be two or more independent disabilities. It may have affected not only complex behaviours like language or cognition, but also motor abilities (cerebral palsy) or have caused epilepsy. No one would disagree with the label 'comorbidity' in combined cerebral palsy and intellectual disability, or epilepsy and language disorder. Despite having a common underlying cause, be it a genetic malformation or acquired brain lesion, each of these disorders can exist in isolation; cerebral palsy, epilepsy and impaired cognition reflect dysfunction in distinct brain circuitry, and they require distinct medical and educational interventions.

The comorbid label is more controversial when the child's particular brain disorder/ maldevelopment (in the singular) affects several of the distributed networks that underlie complex human abilities, to each of which we have given a specific 'diagnosis', which is to say that we have assigned each one to a separate 'pigeon hole'. In contrast to the clearly distinct disorders just invoked, disorders of complex abilities have fuzzy margins and may even be inter-related. A good example is attention-deficit disorder and dyslexia (Shaywitz et al. 1995). We think of such complex disorders as distinct, but it is likely that attention-deficit disorder contributes to the severity of dyslexia or jeopardises its remediation. What we tend to do in such cases is to label the child with the most salient disorder or the one that requires the most intensive or specialised rehabilitation and consider the other(s) comorbid. In Tourette disorder we label as comorbid the regularly associated attention-deficit disorder or executive dysfunction, either of which may create more problems for the child than the tics (Schuerholz et al. 1996). But sometimes we forget that there is actually but one child, with one dysfunctional brain, and that assigning several different 'diagnoses' is a matter of convenience rather than a description of reality.

We also need to remind ourselves that developmental disorders of higher cerebral function are defined dimensionally, and therefore that they have fuzzy margins (Kraemer 1992, Rapin 2002), whereas we created our 'boxes' to sharpen behavioural 'diagnoses', attempting to give the boxes as clear and unambiguous boundaries as possible. Rapid progress in genetics, electrophysiology, imaging and other advanced technologies will soon enable the dichotomous sorting of some of the aetiologies of the developmental disorders yet this will not do away with behavioural comorbidity because what gives rise to the complex overlapping symptomatologies of the developmental disorders is not their cause or aetiology but which inter-related brain systems are dysfunctional. We also need to consider that fuzzy borders mean that there is no sharp partition between personality trait and disorder: the behavioural phenotype deserves to be called a disorder only to the extent that it interferes significantly with everyday life. Both DSM-IV (American Psychiatric Association 2000) and ICD-10 (WHO 1993) make this point, but making the distinction between disorder and personality trait in the less severely affected individual is subjective and likely to lead to disagreement among professionals and parents alike (Nass 2002).

Some individuals with mild disorders militate to be considered different rather than afflicted with a disability (Chamak 2008). Note that fuzziness of behavioural 'diagnoses' results in shifting diagnostic criteria; no doubt this is a main contributor to the current perception of a worldwide ballooning epidemic of autistic spectrum disorders (Wing & Potter 2002, Fombonne 2005).

Some conditions associated with inadequate language development

Unless children have obvious physical signs, epilepsy or motor disabilities, it is often failure to develop language that brings children with a variety of developmental disorders to the attention of parents and professionals. The differential diagnosis is relatively short.

HEARING LOSS

Note first that chronic middle ear effusion or 'glue ear' never produces a hearing loss severe enough to preclude language development, although it may slow the acquisition of phonological precision in speech production, and perhaps the richness of the early lexicon in children with other disabilities or from culturally deprived families (Wallace et al. 1996). Sensorineural hearing loss, especially if it is progressive or high tone, is a hidden disability because the child appears normal in other respects, as non-verbal pragmatics and cognitive development are well developed unless there are comorbidities (Rapin 2006). In fact, hearing loss, whether congenital or later acquired, may be associated with any number of other behaviourally defined comorbidities, including intellectual disability, attention-deficit disorder, autism, reading disability, etc., as well as medical conditions like the long Q-T interval in the electrocardiogram or thyroid dysfunction, to name but two. Hearing loss has readily diagnosable physiological correlates; consequently any child with inadequate language development must forthwith undergo a definitive test of hearing, often including electrophysiology. Missing this disability is a major mistake in that it deprives the child of highly specific and efficacious interventions, the effectiveness of which diminishes with increasing age.

DEVELOPMENTAL LANGUAGE DISORDER (DLD), DYSPHASIA OR SPECIFIC LANGUAGE IMPAIRMENT (SLI))

As with other dimensionally defined developmental disorders, there is no crisp boundary between delayed language and DLD, and no unique diagnostic criterion for DLD. Therefore diagnosis may be made by *exclusionary criteria* – that is, by determining that there is nothing else wrong with the child that might explain the language impairment – or by *positive criteria* – that is, by deviance from expectation for age in reception, processing or production at the levels of phonology (speech sounds), grammar/syntax, semantics (meaning) and/or pragmatics (conversational use) identified clinically and confirmed by a larger or smaller deviation from norms on some standardised test of language. Predictably, different criteria may net vastly different numbers of children as having DLD (Aram et al. 1993).

There is more than one subtype of DLD because language is dependent on such complex cascades of operations. On clinical criteria the two most prevalent are mixed receptive/expressive disorders involving impaired phonological processing, impoverished grammar and semantics, and generally worse production than comprehension, and expressive disorders with preserved comprehension, but there are others (Rapin 1998) which are reasonably congruent with those suggested on the basis of formal analysis of scores on standardised language tests (Conti-Ramsden et al. 1997). It is critical to be aware that there are several different types of developmental language disorders because each requires an individualised rehabilitation approach, whether or not the developmental language disorder is isolated or comorbid with other developmental disorders, including cognitive impairment or autism (American Academy of Child and Adolescent Psychiatry 1998, Tallal et al. 1998, van Weerdenburg et al. 2006).

A major differential diagnostic issue in toddlers and preschoolers is between DLD and DLD comorbid with an autism spectrum disorder. Non-verbal communication (non-verbal pragmatics) is well developed in children with only DLD (Rapin & Dunn 2003). What points to autistic comorbidity is the universally and persistently impaired pragmatics of autism expressed as lack of the drive to compensate for inadequate speech by pointing, nodding, showing, imitating, looking up when called, etc. The speech of verbal children who have an autistic spectrum disorder (ASD) is likely to have atypical or frankly deviant features, listed in Box 5.1. These are red flags that strongly suggest autism although some of them

---

Box 5.1 Features of language suggestive of an autism spectrum disorder

Verbal expression

Impaired pragmatics (communicative use of language), talk to talk rather than
  converse, chatter without communicative intent
Echolalia, persistent pronominal reversal
Scripted utterances (delayed echolalia)
Perseverative questioning
Narrow, repetitive choice of topics, provide too much detail
Esoteric vocabulary; unusual, pedantic word choices
Aberrant prosody:
  sing-song high-pitched voice
  monotonous staccato robotic voice
  rising intonation in assertions

Verbal comprehension

Comprehension paradoxically worse than expression, especially of questions like
  either/or, open-ended what, why, when, how
Lack of awareness of jokes, sarcasm, tone of voice, communicative intent

---

occur in some chatty children with hydrocephalus or Williams syndrome who do not fulfil
the criteria for an ASD.

Besides secondary academic and social comorbid consequences of inadequate communication ability in primary school (Davison & Howlin 1997), severe DLD without autism
puts the older child or adolescent at risk for later school failure and narrows vocational
options, with the result that comorbid social/behavioural problems are frequent (Aram et al.
1984, Stothard et al. 1998).

It is now clear that some three-quarters of children with an inordinate difficulty learning
to read (*dyslexia*) have phonological processing disorder, with or without other deficiencies
(Katzir et al. 2008). Therefore dyslexia is often the later manifestation of the same disorder
that resulted in earlier dysphasia, rather than truly comorbid with DLD. Many, but not all,
older children and adults with dyslexia are in fact 'dysphasic children grown up' whose
difficulty acquiring both oral and written language is due to inadequate phonological processing skills. One can uncover this deficit by asking the child or adult, who now speaks
competently, to read pronounceable non-words or to spell (Bishop 2001). Most individuals
with dyslexia or with 'cured' dyslexia are also slower than expected in automatised word
retrieval (Denckla & Rudel 1976, Grigorenko 2001). As stated earlier, although dyslexia is
often associated with attention-deficit disorder, these are comorbid disorders rather than the
distractibility being the cause of the academic deficit (Shaywitz et al. 1995).

COGNITIVE IMPAIRMENT OR INTELLECTUAL DISABILITY

Intellectual disability (referred to as learning disability, developmental delay or mental retardation in some countries), in contrast to specific developmental disorders like DLD, dyslexia or attention-deficit disorder, refers to inadequacy of multiple skills required to function independently in everyday life (American Psychiatric Association 2000). If intellectual disability is not too severe, gross motor skills may not be affected, so this disability may pass unnoticed for a long time, often until the challenge of school. Moreover, intellectual disability has to be severe to preclude the development of language. A comorbid hearing impairment should also be considered as a contributory factor for speech delay in a child with intellectual impairment.

Milder degrees of intellectual disability are likely to delay the development of both comprehension and production of speech. The question is whether the severity of the language impairment is out of proportion to the severity of the deficit in non-verbal and adaptive skills, in other words out of proportion to the severity of the intellectual disability. When it is, it is appropriate to invoke comorbidity and state that the child is both intellectually disabled and language impaired.

Intellectual disability, like other developmental disorders, has many aetiologies with selective effects on the development of particular brain networks. The huge variety of causes results in disparate behavioural phenotypes, some of which are highly correlated with a particular disorder. Well-known examples are the more severely affected verbal expression of children with Down syndrome (Chapman et al. 1998) and the sparing of expressive language in Williams syndrome (Bellugi et al. 1999, Martens et al. 2008). Severely impaired language comprehension, with consequently inadequate expression, will lower the full scale IQ score, in some cases into the borderline or mildly intellectually impaired range. This emphasises why a detailed neuropsychological inventory is so important in developmentally impaired children, as it is likely to yield a much more detailed and informative cognitive profile and potential than the full-scale IQ to guide educational remediation.

AUTISM (AUTISM SPECTRUM DISORDERS (ASD), PERVASIVE DEVELOPMENTAL DISORDERS (PDD))

It is regularly either failure to develop language or regression of what language the toddler or preschool child had developed that brings the child to parental and professional attention (Wilson et al. 2003). Unfortunately professionals all too often falsely reassure parents, which delays the provision of appropriate remedial education. The language disorders of autism overlap those of children with DLD, but with some differences (see Box 5.1) (Rapin & Dunn 2003). Developmental language disorders are one of the core deficits of autism. It is not the case that either the social disabilities or the intellectual disability account adequately for the language deficits of children with autism. MRI morphometry shows that groups of children with ASD and DLD with language subtypes characterised by inadequate expressive phonology have reversed asymmetry of Broca's area in common (de Fossé et al. 2004) and that the volume of the left superior temporal gyrus is not correlated with receptive language ability in autism as it is in non-autistic dyslexic controls, interpreted as inadequate lateralisation for language in the autism group (Bigler et al. 2007). Although these small studies require replication, they suggest that the language deficits in children with autism and with DLD denote dysfunction of overlapping circuitry, in other words that the language deficits parallel those of DLD, albeit with differences in base rates. Although high-functioning individuals with autism may eventually speak well, and by definition those with Asperger syndrome were not delayed in expressive language acquisition, they nonetheless retain life-long deficits in some language skills (Tager-Flusberg 2003).

Pragmatics, that is, the communicative use of language, is uniquely and invariably inadequate and remains so throughout life in individuals on the autistic spectrum, albeit with altered and often more subtle signs of impairment than in early childhood. Some of the tell-tale signs are not looking up when called by name, difficulty initiating and maintaining conversation, rigidity in choice of topic, perseveration such as incessant questioning, parroting (immediate echolalia) and use of scripts (formulaic speech), unusual word choices, aberrant prosody and gaze avoidance. *Prosody*, the rhythm and melody of speech, is often deviant, the voice high-pitched or singsong, assertions having the rising intonation of questions, and rhythm being choppy or wooden.

At early ages, *comprehension* is invariably affected. In fact, it may be more compromised than expression in fluent children who may have a large oversophisticated vocabulary and speak better than they understand discourse (connected speech). Inability to answer questions because of failure to master question forms at the expected age is a sign of impaired comprehension. Inadequate comprehension is easily brought out by the children's difficulty in answering questions and their chaining to words rather than ideas and therefore straying off topic. *Syntax and phonology* (grammar and speech sounds) may or may not be affected (Rapin et al. 2009) whereas, at least in young children, *semantics* (meaning of words and discourse) is invariably deficient.

In some children, phonology – and therefore all subsequent language decoding/encoding operations – is so severely compromised as to render the child totally uncomprehending and mute, and in some cases permanently so (verbal auditory agnosia – VAA) (Kaga 1999). If children with this most severe receptive/expressive disorder do acquire some expressive language, it will be, and may remain, poorly articulated and dysfluent, with impoverished syntax and vocabulary, as well as inadequate pragmatics and limited comprehension. Bear in mind that non-verbal children with rare well-articulated utterances do not have VAA and may unaccountably start to express themselves verbally and intelligibly, usually before age 5 years, and rarely even later.

A HITHERTO SILENT EARLY LATERALISED BRAIN LESION

Lateralised hemispheric lesions acquired *in utero* or in the first year of life, most often a stroke in the middle cerebral artery territory, present as delayed, not aberrant language acquisition (Bates 1999). This is true whether the lesion was in the left or the right (Ballantyne et al. 2007) – so much for the idea that language is the affair of only the left hemisphere! Such children can confidently be expected to develop adequate language, provided the contralateral hemisphere is unaffected. This contrasts with lateralised (predominantly left) brain lesions sustained by older children who have already acquired language: their aphasias follow quite closely the acquired aphasic syndromes of adults (van Hout 1997). Whether in infants with lateralised lesions language will pre-empt other portions of the left hemisphere or shift to the contralateral right hemisphere depends on how much of the perisylvian cortex has been destroyed by the early lesion (Milner 1974). Contralateral shift is especially likely if the original lesion involved Broca's inferior frontal area which is critical for expressive language. A comparison of children with left and right perisylvian lesions may reveal subtle language differences, with left lesions having a greater effect on phonology and syntax and right lesions on vocabulary (Aram et al. 1985) although, contrary to expectation, very early lesions in anterior versus posterior cortical language areas do not have differential effects on expression and comprehension of language (Bates 1999). Subcortical lesions affecting the basal ganglia or internal capsule tend to have more lasting effects on expressive language than cortical lesions (Aram et al. 1983).

Contrary to what is widely believed, recovery from acquired aphasia in childhood is rarely complete even though oral language is regained, as deficits in the acquisition of written language, mathematics and other academic skills, and subtle personality difficulties are frequent (Nass & Trauner 2004). The price to pay for aberrant development of language in the right hemisphere is frequent 'crowding out' of other skills, classically visuospatial skills, an often overlooked neuropsychological comorbidity (Stiles et al. 2003).

It is important to differentiate *dysarthria* or *anarthria* from a severe expressive language deficit that may be either isolated (verbal dyspraxia) (Hayden 1994) or associated with a generally less severe receptive deficit (mixed receptive/expressive dysphasia). Dysarthria may be due to bilateral corticobulbar pathology (pseudo-bulbar palsy), the choreo-athetosis of basal ganglia lesions or severe cerebellar pathology. What distinguishes dysarthria from verbal dyspraxia is impairment of voluntary movements of the face, mastication, swallowing and phonation. These oromotor deficits are much more severely affected in dysarthria than in verbal dyspraxia or mixed receptive/expressive dysphasia, although lesser degrees of dysarthria are quite often, but by no means always, comorbid in the mixed or expressive dysphasias.

Fortunately usually reversible and unique to childhood, surgical procedures that involve the cerebellar vermis are in some cases followed by mutism, often associated with social withdrawal akin to autism (Riva & Giorgi 2000). This is highly relevant in view of the well-documented cerebellar pathology of autism (Bauman & Kemper 2005, Courchesne et al. 1988).

SELECTIVE MUTISM

This refers to failure to speak, usually with adequate comprehension, which may be very long-lasting but is situationally related, such as mutism in school or outside the home, with by report normal expression at home. This is a dangerous diagnosis to make unless there is documentation by a competent observer or, better, on video- or audiotape, that the child's language is adequate in some environments. Some children with selective mutism have comorbidities such as DLD, autism, anxiety or depression (Steinhausen & Juzi 1996).

Comorbidity in language regression

Regression of previously acquired language of unknown cause in the absence of a documented brain lesion or degenerative disease of the brain occurs in childhood in the following, in some cases overlapping, disorders.

ACQUIRED EPILEPTIC APHASIA (LANDAU–KLEFFNER SYNDROME (LKS))

Regression usually occurs between 3 and 6 years, rarely earlier or later, and by definition takes place in the context of either clinical seizures or an epileptiform EEG without clinical seizures (subclinical epilepsy) (Dugas et al. 1991). It is due to a severe or total deficit in the ability to process language by ear – VAA, which in children results in prompt regression of expressive language (speech) (Rapin et al. 1977). First brought to medical attention in 1957 (Landau & Kleffner 1957), this rare disorder typically is not associated with inadequate non-verbal pragmatics, frank autistic features or dementia, although it may engender behavioural abnormalities such as frustration, depression or some other reactive behavioural response to the inability to communicate. There is considerable debate, however, regarding the boundaries of LKS and its overlaps with other epileptic and developmental disorders of childhood, including autistic regression (Stefanatos et al. 2002, Tuchman & Rapin 2002) and electrical status epilepticus in slow-wave sleep (ESES) (Nickels & Wirrell 2008).

The language deficit in LKS is specific to the auditory channel, which means that the children are capable of acquiring/processing language visually. In the vast majority of cases, LKS affects phonological decoding (VAA) but early in the course of severe cases it may result in cortical deafness (Kaga 1999). Rare cases with predominantly expressive deficits have been reported. LKS overlaps developmental VAA which was first described in the 19th century (Worster-Drought & Allen 1930). Developmental VAA is the most severe DLD because children may be rendered essentially uncomprehending and non-verbal. Contrary to acquired LKS, developmental VAA may or may not be associated with clinical or subclinical epilepsy (Klein et al. 2000).

The seizures in acquired LKS are of various types, often, but by no means always, complex partial (Tuchman et al. 1991). The EEG epileptiform activity involves perisylvian cortex either bilaterally or unilaterally on the right or the left, and is activated by slow-wave sleep (McVicar & Shinnar 2004). The seizures almost always subside before adolescence, with/without antiepileptic drugs, but the language may or may not improve. The MRI is usually uninformative although morphometry may reveal superior temporal lobe atrophy (Takeoka et al. 2004).

The epileptiform activity in LKS has many similarities to Rolandic epilepsy or benign epilepsy of childhood with centrotemporal spikes (BECTS) (Massa et al. 2000); whether LKS and BECTS are distinct or one disorder with differing severities is unclear. Rolandic epilepsy may interfere transiently with speech and is also limited to childhood. The cause of both remains undetermined but has genetic implications (Rudolf et al. 2009). Searching neuropsychological testing may uncover some mild persistent cognitive deficits (Piccinelli et al. 2008), but rolandic epilepsy never renders children non-verbal, whereas LKS frequently does. As in LKS, the epileptiform EEG activity in rolandic activity is much more

82

active than one would predict from the clinical seizures and is also enhanced in slow-wave sleep (Kramer 2008). The source of the epileptiform activity involves auditory/language perisylvian cortical language areas in LKS, with a left preponderance, whereas in children on the autistic spectrum who regress there tends to be, in addition, more widespread epileptiform activity (Lewine et al. 1999).

AUTISTIC/LANGUAGE REGRESSION

Here the regression occurs earlier (usually between 18 and 24 months) than in LKS and it is not limited to language but also involves joint attention, non-verbal pragmatics, imaginative play and in some cases cognition, but essentially never motor skills (Shinnar et al. 2001, Wilson et al. 2003). Regression is reported by parents and sometimes documented on videos in previously normally developing children or in children who, if they already had autistic symptomatology, were less severely affected than following the regression (Luyster et al. 2005).

Autistic/language regression is associated with clinical or subclinical epilepsy in only some 10% of cases (Tuchman & Rapin 1997). Such cases are considered by some investigators to represent a broader form of LKS (Stefanatos et al. 2002). Whether this is a heuristic point of view remains to be determined. Although parents attribute the regression to a variety of triggers, none, including epilepsy, is a proven aetiology. As it has been shown that multigenic inheritance is the most prevalent cause of autism, perhaps in some cases one or more of the inherited genes enhances vulnerability to some environmental, generally innocuous circumstance that might trigger the regression (Schanen 2006). This plausible hypothesis has not been validated by data, immunological or otherwise, so that it is no more than a speculation at present.

DISINTEGRATIVE DISORDER

According to DSM-IV/ICD-10, disintegrative disorder refers to loss of speech, social skills and often cognition to the point of frank dementia, following fully normal early development and language, and it is not due to a degenerative disease of the brain (Hendry 2000). It is very much rarer than autism (Fombonne 2002), overlaps with delayed autistic regression, and it is not clear whether these are truly separate disorders (Malhotra & Gupta 1999). In most cases the child becomes non-verbal and remains so. Prognosis is guarded as improvement is less likely than in early autistic regression. Disintegrative disorder may or may not be associated with clinical/subclinical epilepsy, including ESES (Rapin 1995). It is more important than in infantile autism to consider an insidiously progressive underlying brain disease which may not be evident for years, because the yield for one is probably considerably higher than in early regression.

RETT SYNDROME

This disorder is due, in some 80% of cases, to one of several mutations in the *MEPC2* gene on Xq33 (Amir et al. 1999). In most cases its phenotype is salient enough for a reliable clinical diagnosis because the postnatal stagnation of brain growth, regression in sociability, irritability, often continuous hand stereotypies, later epilepsy and other physical signs that appear in the first or second year after fully normal early development (Kerr et al. 2001) are distinctive. Most of the children are entirely non-verbal or minimally verbal and many do not achieve ambulation. It is now known that the phenotype is broader than previously thought in females (Hagberg & Gillberg 1993) and that very severely affected males are encountered (Moog et al. 2003).

SOME OTHER INSIDIOUSLY PROGRESSIVE GENETIC/METABOLIC BRAIN DISEASES

Each of these conditions is extremely rare but all may be associated with impaired language development or its regression. All of them have tell-tale evidence of an ongoing neurological condition, usually epilepsy and motor deficits, and other more specific signs that assist in narrowing diagnostic possibilities. The few mentioned below are but a sample of those to consider, especially in children whose course is one of slowing, followed by arrest of developmental progress, and then decay of previous abilities, especially language and cognition. The remote possibility of such a disorder calls for the longitudinal evaluation of all children with developmental disorders by one physician who is less likely to overlook deterioration than parents or professionals who see the child on a daily basis or physicians who only see the child cross-sectionally. Most of these disorders have several clinical and genetic variants and require evaluation by neurologists and geneticists with expertise in this type of disorder. Some of the disorders without salient physical findings to consider include Sanfilippo type III, neuroaxonal dystrophy, ceroid lipofuscinosis with/without visual loss and malignant epileptic encephalopathies of early childhood like Lennox–Gastaut syndrome, and many others.

Conclusion

Inadequate language development or language loss is a feature of many developmental and acquired disorders of the immature brain. It is often impaired language that brings the child to professional attention, therefore it is not a parental complaint to dismiss lightly despite the wide variability in the milestones and styles of early language acquisition (Bates et al. 1994). The possibility of a hearing loss needs to be at the forefront of the differential diagnosis unless the child's language is fluent and well articulated, in which case consideration shifts from a disorder that affects auditory processing of language (phonology) to a disorder of higher order language processing, cognition or social skills, notably an autistic spectrum disorder. The four most likely conditions to consider are hearing loss, intellectual disability, specific language disorder and an autistic spectrum disorder. Detailed family histories and background histories of the child's development and health, together with the neurological evaluation, will guide how extensively one needs to consider the possibility of an underlying structural brain lesion, epilepsy or an obscure genetic condition. In the absence of any clinical clue, massive work-ups for such conditions which are not hypothesis driven are generally wasteful, stressful, expensive and unwarranted unless they are performed in the context of a formal research project. On the other hand, longitudinal follow-up is essential to keep physicians on the alert for a rare disorder with medical implications. Mendelian or mitochondrial gene defects and cytogenetic abnormalities have implications for genetic counselling, but genetic deficits discovered by microarray analysis essentially never have medical implications for the child, and definite implications for genetic counselling are rare, at least at our present level of knowledge, and especially in view of the extreme phenotypic variability of developmental disorders.

To whatever 'diagnostic box' the child is assigned, language comorbidity requires specific intervention. This intervention is usually more effective if provided in an intensive educational setting that addresses each of the child's specific rehabilitative needs. Children who are non-verbal, whether or not they are also uncomprehending, require assistive communicative devices, be they gestures, Sign, pictures or computers. The ability to communicate one's needs and ideas is so fundamental to human welfare that attention to providing a channel for language, however primitive it may seem, is an essential part of the rehabilitation of all children with any developmental disorder.

REFERENCES

American Academy of Child and Adolescent Psychiatry (1998) Summary of the practice parameters for the assessment and treatment of children and adolescents with language and learning disorders. *J Am Acad Child Adolesc Psychiatr* **37**(10), 1117–1119.

American Psychiatric Association (2000) *Diagnostic and Statistical Manual of Mental Disorders,* 4th edn, revised. Washington, DC: American Psychiatric Association.

Amir RE, van den Veyver IB, Wan M, Tran CQ, Francke U, Zoghbi HY (1999) Rett syndrome is caused by mutations in x-linked *MECP2*, encoding methyl-CpG-binding protein. *Nat Genet* **23**(10), 185–188.

Aram DM, Rose DF, Rekate HL,Whitaker HA (1983) Acquired capsular/striatal aphasia in childhood. *Arch Neurol* **40**(10), 614–617.

Aram DM, Ekelman BL, Nation JE (1984) Preschoolers with language disorders: 10 years later. *J Speech Hear Res* **27**(2), 232–244.

Aram DM, Ekelman BL, Rose DF, Whitaker HA (1985) Verbal and cognitive sequelae following unilateral lesions acquired in early childhood. *J Clin Exper Neuropsychol* **7**(1), 55–78.

Aram DM, Morris R, Hall NE (1993) Clinical and research congruence in identifying children with specific language impairment. *J Speech Hear Res* **36**(3), 580–591.

Ballantyne AO, Spilkin AM, Trauner DA (2007) Language outcome after perinatal stroke: does side matter? *Child Neuropsychol* **13**(6), 494–509.

Bates E (1999) Plasticity, localization and language development. In: Broman SH, Fletcher J (eds) *The Changing Nervous System: Neurobehavioral Consequences of Early Brain Development.* New York: Oxford University Press, pp. 214–253.

Bates E, Marchman V, Thal D, et al. (1994) Developmental and stylistic variation in the composition of early vocabulary *J Child Lang* **21**(1), 85–123.

Bauman ML, Kemper TL (2005) Neuroanatomic observations of the brain in autism: a review and future directions. *Int J Dev Neurosci* **23**(2–3), 183–187.

Bellugi U, Lichtenberger L, Mills D, Galaburda A, Korenberg JR (1999) Bridging cognition, the brain and molecular genetics: evidence from Williams syndrome. *Trends Neurosci* **22**(5), 197–207.

Bigler ED, Mortensen S, Neeley ES, et al. (2007) Superior temporal gyrus, language function, and autism. *Dev Neuropsychol* **31**(2), 217–238.

Bishop DV (2001) Genetic influences on language impairment and literacy problems in children: same or different? *J Child Psychol Psychiatr* **42**(2), 189–198.

Chamak B (2008) Autism and social movements: French parents associations and international autistic individuals organisations. *Sociol Health Illness* **30**, 76–96.

Chapman RS, Seung HK, Schwartz SE, Kay-Raining Bird E (1998) Language skills of children and adolescents with Down syndrome: II. Production deficits. *J Speech Lang Hear Res* **41**(4), 861–873.

Conti-Ramsden G, Crutchley A, Botting N (1997) The extent to which psychometric tests differentiate subgroups of children with SLI. *J Speech Lang Hear Res* **40**(4), 765–777.

Courchesne E, Yeung-Courchesne R, Press GA, Hesselink JR, Jernigan TL (1988) Hypoplasia of cerebellar vermal lobules VI and VII in autism. *N Engl J Med* **318**(21), 1349–1354.

Davison FM, Howlin P (1997) A follow-up study of children attending a primary-age language unit. *Eur J Disord Commun* **32**(1), 19–36.

De Fosse L, Hodge SM, Makris N, et al. (2004) Language-association cortex asymmetry in autism and specific language impairment. *Ann Neurol* **56**(6), 757–766.

Denckla MB, Rudel RG (1976) Rapid automatized naming (R.A.N): dyslexia differentiated from other learning disabilities. *Neuropsychologia* **14**(4), 471–479.

Dugas M, Gerard CL, Franc S, Sagar D (1991) Natural history, course and prognosis of the Landau and Kleffner syndrome. In: Pavao Martins I, et al. (eds) *Acquired Aphasia in Children: Acquisition and Breakdown of Language in the Developing Brain*. Dordrecht: Kluwer Academic, pp. 263–277.

Fombonne E (2002) Prevalence of childhood disintegrative disorder. *Autism* **6**(2), 149–157.

Fombonne E (2005) Epidemiology of autistic disorder and other pervasive developmental disorders. *J Clin Psychiatr* **66**(Suppl 10), 3–8.

Grigorenko EL (2001) Developmental dyslexia: an update on genes, brains, and environments. *J Child Psychol Psychiatr Allied Disc* **42**(1), 91–125.

Hagberg B, Gillberg C (1993) Rett variants – Rettoid phenotypes. In: Hagberg B (ed) *Rett Syndrome – Clinical and Biological Aspects*. London: Mac Keith Press, pp. 40–60.

Hayden DA (1994) Differential diagnosis of motor speech dysfunction in children. *Clin Commun Disord* **4**(2),119–141.

Hendry CN (2000) Childhood disintegrative disorder: should it be considered a distinct diagnosis? *Clin Psychol Rev* **20**(1), 77–90.

Kaga M (1999) Language disorders in Landau–Kleffner syndrome. *J Child Neurol* **14**, 118–122.

Katzir T, Kim YS, Wolf M, Morris R, Lovett MW (2008) The varieties of pathways to dysfluent reading: comparing subtypes of children with dyslexia at letter, word, and connected text levels of reading. *J Learning Disabil* **41**(1), 47–66.

Kerr AM, Nomura Y, Armstrong D, et al. (2001) Guidelines for reporting clinical features in cases with MECP2 mutations. *Brain Dev.* **23**(4), 208–211.

Klein SK, Tuchman RF, Rapin I (2000) The influence of premorbid language skills and behavior on language recovery in children with verbal auditory agnosia. *J Child Neurol* **15**(1), 36–43.

Kraemer HC (1992) Measurement of reliability for categorical data in medical research. *Stat Methods Med Res* **1**, 183–199.

Kramer U (2008) Atypical presentations of benign childhood epilepsy with centrotemporal spikes: a review. *J Child Neurol* **23**(7), 785–790.

Landau WM, Kleffner FR (1957) Syndrome of acquired aphasia with convulsive disorder in children. *Neurology* **7**, 523–530.

Lewine JD, Andrews R, Chez M, et al. (1999) Magnetoencephalographic patterns of epileptiform activity in children with regressive autism spectrum disorders. *Pediatrics* **104**(3 Pt 1), 405–418.

Luyster R, Richler J, Risi S, et al. (2005) Early regression in social communication in autism spectrum disorders: a CPEA study. *Dev Neuropsychol* **27**(3), 311–336.

Malhotra S, Gupta N (1999) Childhood disintegrative disorder. *J Autism Dev Disord* **29**(6), 491–498.

Martens MA, Wilson SJ, Reutens DC (2008) Research review: Williams syndrome: a critical review of the cognitive, behavioral, and neuroanatomical phenotype. *J Child Psychol Psychiatr Allied Disc* **49**(6), 576–608.

Massa R, Saint-Martin A, Hirsch E (2000) Landau–Kleffner syndrome: sleep EEG characteristics at onset. *Clin.Neurophysiol* **111**(Suppl 2), S87–S93.

McVicar KA, Shinnar S (2004) Landau–Kleffner syndrome, electrical status epilepticus in sleep, and language regression in children. *Mental Retard Dev Disabil Res Rev* **10**(2), 144–149.

Milner B (1974) Hemispheric specialization: scope and limits. In: Schmitt FO, Worden FG (eds) *The Neurosciences. Third Study Program*. Cambridge, MA: MIT Press, pp. 75–89.

Moog U, Smeets EE, van Roozendaal Ke, et al. (2003) Neurodevelopmental disorders in males related to the gene causing Rett syndrome in females (MECP2). *Eur J Paediatr Neurol* **7**(1), 5–12.

Nass R (2002) Plasticity: mechanisms, extent and limits. In: Segalowitz SJ, Rapin I (eds) *Child Neuropsychology*, 2nd edn. Amsterdam: Elsevier, pp. 29–68.

Nass RD, Trauner D (2004) Social and affective impairments are important to recovery after acquired stroke in childhood. *CNS Spectrums* **9**(6), 420–434.

Nickels K, Wirrell E (2008) Electrical status epilepticus in sleep. *Semin Pediatr Neurol* **15**(2), 50–60.

Piccinelli P, Borgatti R, Aldini A, et al. (2008) Academic performance in children with rolandic epilepsy. *Dev Med Child Neurol* **50**(5), 353–356.

Rapin I (1995) Autistic regression and disintegrative disorder: how important is the role of epilepsy? *Semin Pediatr Neurol* **4**, 278–285.

Rapin I (1998) Understanding childhood language disorders. *Curr Opin Pediatr* **10**(6), 561–566.

Rapin I (2002) Diagnostic dilemmas in developmental disabilities: fuzzy margins at the edges of normality. An essay prompted by Thomas Sowell's new book: *The Einstein Syndrome. J Autism Dev Disord* **32**(1), 49–57.

Rapin I (2006) Hearing impairment. In: Swaiman KF, Ashwal S, Ferriero DM (eds) *Pediatric Neurology*, 4th edn. St Louis, MI: Mosby, pp. 97–122.

Rapin I, Dunn M (2003) Update on the language disorders of individuals on the autistic spectrum. *Brain Dev* **25**(3), 166–172.

Rapin I, Mattis S, Rowan AJ, Golden GS (1977) Verbal auditory agnosia in children. *Dev Med Child Neurol* **19**, 192–207.

Rapin I, Dunn M, Allen DA, Stevens M, Fein D (2009) Subtypes of language disorders in schoolage children with autism. *Dev Neuropsychol* **34**(1), 1–9.

Riva D, Giorgi C (2000) The cerebellum contributes to higher functions during development: evidence from a series of children surgically treated for posterior fossa tumours. *Brain* **123**(Pt 5), 1051–1061.

Rudolf G, Valenti MP, Hirsch E, Szepetowski P (2009) From rolandic epilepsy to continuous spike-and-waves during sleep and Landau–Kleffner syndromes: insights into possible genetic factors. *Epilepsia* **50** (Suppl 7), 25–28.

Schanen NC (2006) Epigenetics of autism spectrum disorders. *Hum Mol Genet* **15**(2), R138–R150.

Schuerholz LJ, Baumgardner TL, Singer HS, Reiss AL, Denckla MB (1996) Neuropsychological status of children with Tourette's syndrome with and without attention deficit hyperactivity disorder. *Neurology* **46**(4), 958–965.

Shaywitz BA, Fletcher JM, Shaywitz SE (1995) Defining and classifying learning disabilities and attention-deficit/hyperactivity disorder. *J Child Neurol* **10**(Suppl 1), S50–S57.

Shinnar S, Rapin I, Arnold S, et al. (2001) Language regression in childhood. *Pediatric Neurol* **24**(3), 185–191.

Stefanatos GA, Kinsbourne M, Wasserstein J (2002) Acquired epileptiform aphasia: a dimensional view of Landau–Kleffner syndrome and the relation to regressive autistic spectrum disorders *Child Neuropsychol* **8**(3), 195–228.

Steinhausen HC, Juzi C (1996) Elective mutism: an analysis of 100 cases. *J Am Acad Child Adolesc Psychiatr* **35**(5), 606–614.

Stiles J, Moses P, Roe K, et al. (2003) Alternative brain organization after prenatal cerebral injury: convergent fMRI and cognitive data. *J Int Neuropsychol Soc* **9**(4), 604–622.

Stothard SE, Snowling MJ, Bishop DVM, Chipchase BB, Kaplan CA (1998) Language-impaired preschoolers: a follow-up into adolescence. *J Speec Lang Hear Res* **41**, 407–418.

Tager-Flusberg H (2003) Language impairments in children with complex neurodevelopmental disorders: the case of autism. In: Levy Y, Schaeffer J (eds) *Language Competence Across Populations: Toward a Definition of Specific Language Impairment.* Mahwah, NJ: Lawrence Erlbaum Associates, pp. 297–321.

Takeoka M, Riviello JJ Jr, Duffy FH, et al. (2004) Bilateral volume reduction of the superior temporal areas in Landau–Kleffner syndrome. *Neurology* **63**(7), 1289–1292.

Tallal P, Merzenich MM, Miller S, Jenkins W (1998) Language learning impairments: integrating basic science, technology, and remediation. *Exper Brain Res* **123**(1-2), 210–219.

Tuchman RF, Rapin I (1997) Regression in pervasive developmental disorders: seizures and epileptiform EEG correlates. *Pediatrics* **99**(4), 560–566.

Tuchman RF, Rapin I (2002) Epilepsy in autism. *Lancet Neurol* **1**, 352–358.

Tuchman RF, Rapin I, Shinnar S (1991) Autistic and dysphasic children: II. Epilepsy, *Pediatrics* **88**(6), 1219–1225.

van Hout A (1997) Acquired aphasia in children. *Semin Pediatr Neurol* **4**(2), 102–108.

van Weerdenburg M, Verhoeven L, van Balkom H (2006) Towards a typology of specific language impairment. *J Child Psychol Psychiatr Allied Disc* **47**(2), 176–189.

Wallace IF, Gravel JS, Schwartz RG, Ruben RJ (1996) Otitis media, communication style of primary caregivers, and language skills of 2 year olds: a preliminary report. *J Dev Behav Pediatr* **17**(1), 27–35.

Wilson S, Djukic A, Shinnar S, Dharmani C, Rapin I (2003) Clinical characteristics of language regression in children. *Dev Med Child Neurol* **45**, 508–514.

Wing L, Potter D (2002) The epidemiology of autistic spectrum disorders: is the prevalence rising? *Mental Retard Dev Disabil Res Rev* **8**(3), 151–161.

World Health Organization (1993) *Mental Disorders: Glossary and Guide to their Classification in Accordance with the Tenth Revision of the International Classification of Diseases.* Geneva: World Health Organization.

Worster-Drought C, Allen IM (1930) Congenital auditory imperception (congenital word-deafness): and its relation to idioglossia and other speech defects. *J Neurol Psychopatho* **10**, 193–236.

6
AUTISM AND EPILEPSY: COMORBIDITY, COEXISTENCE OR COINCIDENCE?

Christopher Gillberg and Brian Neville

Many individuals with autism have epilepsy and many of those with epilepsy have autism. In 1908, Theodor Heller described a condition that he referred to as 'dementia infantilis' which is now considered an autism spectrum disorder. The rate of epilepsy in this rare disorder is extremely high. In 1932, Critchley and Earl described the coexistence of epilepsy and the condition that we currently refer to as autism in the 'neurocutaneous' disorder categorised as tuberous sclerosis (or Bourneville disease), and which we now know to be caused by genetic lesions on either chromosome 9 or chromosome 16. In 1943, Kanner described 11 children with his then new 'autistic disturbances of affective contact'. One of these 11 suffered from epilepsy. In 1971, Kanner reported on a follow-up of the 11 patients; by now, two patients (18% of his original series) were suffering from epilepsy. Thus, in this seminal report, which defined autism, the patients already formed a clinically hetero-geneous group – those with and those without seizures.

What has become clear over the years since Kanner's writings is that patients with autism are, in fact, at greater risk of seizures than are children with other types of develop-mental problems, such as developmental dysphasia or Down syndrome (Wong 1993). The frequency of epilepsy in autism, regardless of intelligence quotient (IQ), is higher than in 'non-autism' severe intellectual disability (Gillberg et al. 1986), even though a population of individuals with severe intellectual disability is likely to include a fraction with autism (often with a diagnosable genetic 'double' syndrome).

Prevalence of epilepsy in autism and of autism in epilepsy
The variation in reported percentage of epilepsy in a group of individuals with autism is best explained by the fact that we are dealing with a set of syndromes – a collection of different diseases and disorders that share a distinctive pattern of behaviour. Some disease/disorder entities within the 'autisms' are seizure free; others have many, but not all, indi-viduals who suffer from epilepsy. Both patients with 'classic autism' (with classic symp-tomatology and, as yet, no established syndromal or aetiological/pathogenetic link) and those with double syndromes (autism with another known 'non-epilepsy' medical disorder) may suffer from epilepsy. The latter group includes cases with Angelman syndrome, Rett syndrome, fragile X syndrome, tuberous sclerosis, sex chromosome aneuploidies, Landau–Kleffner syndrome, Smith–Lemli–Opitz syndrome, Smith–Magenis syndrome, Sanfilippo A and phenylketonuria, among many others.

If one looks at studies of individuals with autism, the percentage of those with epilepsy varies greatly. The prevalence of epilepsy in the general population is 0.5%; the published figures on epilepsy in autism range from 4% to 47% (Carod et al. 1995). There appear to be at least two reasons for this rather large variation. One is the fact that each group of patients with autism contains a different mixture of disease entities within the whole, some of which have seizures and some of which do not. Secondly, the frequency of epilepsy varies with the length of the follow-up period, rising as the follow-up period lengthens. Although epilepsy in children with autism often appears during the first 3 years of life (Ritvo et al. 1990), new cases emerge through childhood, adolescence and into adult life (Danielsson et al. 2005). The rate of epilepsy in autism tends to be highest in general population samples of cases with autism followed from childhood into adult life, and lowest in child and adolescent psychiatric clinic patients with autism looked at cross-sectionally at any time under 18 years of age.

Also, individuals with 'classic' autism usually have varying degrees of intellectual disability, and the rate of epilepsy is higher in those with lower IQ. Thus, if one considers the rate of epilepsy only in those with classic autism, the percentage is about 35% (Billstedt et al. 2005). In those with other types of autism 'spectrum' disorders, including Asperger syndrome, the rate is considerably lower, probably of the order of 5–15%. Thus, if one were to suggest an epilepsy prevalence rate for all the autisms (including cases with intellectual disability and cases with low-normal, normal or above-average IQ), it would probably be in the range of 10–20%. The one study that has looked at the prevalence of epilepsy in high-functioning cases (a study of 100 young males with Asperger syndrome) found that 7% had the combination of Asperger syndrome and epilepsy (Cederlund et al. 2008).

An epidemiological study of infantile autism conducted in a county in Norway found that out of 28 persons with autism, nine (32%) had epilepsy (Herder 1993). In a Spanish series of 62 children with autism (Carod et al. 1995), 47% had some kind of epileptic syndrome, including two children with brain tumours, which is an unusual finding in any autism series. Danielsson et al. (2008) and Billstedt et al. (2005), in their Swedish general population cohort of 120 individuals with classic autism (n=87) and atypical autism (n=33), found that a full 40% had developed epilepsy in early adult life. Billstedt et al. (2007), reporting from the same cohort, found that mortality was very high in autism (8% had died between ages 10 and 40 years) and that much of the increased mortality rate was attributable to epilepsy (including several cases of sudden unexplained death in epilepsy).

Autism is extremely common in epilepsy, particularly when there is associated intellectual disability (Steffenburg et al. 1996). About half of all individuals with the combination of autism and learning disability have either autistic disorder or another autistic-like condition. The situation is further complicated by the fact that children with the triad of epilepsy, intellectual disability and autism very often also meet full criteria for attention-deficit–hyperactivity disorder.

Gender aspects
Wing (1981) suggested early on that girls diagnosed with autism have more severe indices of brain damage than boys, this being one of the reasons why they are over-represented

at very low IQ levels. Danielsson et al. (2008) found that girls with autism were relatively much more likely than boys to suffer from epilepsy. In a large American series of 302 children with autism, Tuchman et al. (1991) reported that epilepsy occurred in 14%. In this series, girls were affected more frequently than boys (24% versus 11%). (When cognitive and motor disabilities were excluded, the risk of epilepsy in children with autism was only 6%.) Elia et al. (1995) also found that females were more frequently affected by seizures than males in an Italian series of individuals with autism and intellectual disability.

A review and meta-analysis of all published reports 1963–2006 of epilepsy in autism concluded that females are at relatively much higher risk of the combination of epilepsy and autism than are males, and that epilepsy is much more common (21%) in children with autism and intellectual disability than in those with normal levels of intelligence (8%) (Amiet et al. 2008). Nevertheless, there was a much higher rate of epilepsy in the more high-functioning group as well (8% versus 0.5% in the general population), indicating a strong link between autism 'per se' and epilepsy (our conclusion).

Diagnostic/differential diagnostic aspects including electroencephalogram
Standard electroencephalograms (EEGs) are helpful when they reveal frankly epileptiform activity (Rapin 1997). Based on a review of the medical literature up to that time, Tsai et al. (1985) reported that the majority of children with autism have shown some kind of EEG abnormality whether they had seizures or not. However, if the abnormal EEG readings are limited to epileptiform findings, this figure declines. Rossi et al. (1995) examined 106 patients with autism and found that 23.6% had paroxysmal EEG abnormalities compared to 18.9% with actual clinical seizures. Chez et al. (2006), reporting on the largest autism-EEG cohort to date (n=889), found that 61% had epileptiform activity during sleep, in spite of having no diagnosed clinical seizure disorder.

When one looks at the picture from the public health point of view of how much epilepsy and intellectual disability exist in a general population, there is the additional question of how much autism contributes to this cohort. An answer has been given by a population-based study of 6–13 year olds which identified 98 children with active epilepsy and intellectual disability and reported that an autistic disorder was present in 27% and an autistic-like disorder in 11% of these children (Steffenburg et al. 1995).

AUTISTIC REGRESSION AND EPILEPSY
About a third of toddlers with autism appear to regress in language, sociability, play and often cognition (Rapin 1995). Some of this is probably not due to 'real' regression but is produced by the fact that children who develop 'normally' for about 18 months or so thereafter do not have the communication 'building blocks' to develop more complex forms of language and cognition, and hence stop using what little language they may have had. The studies by Billstedt et al. (2007) and Fernell et al. (2010) suggest that only about one in 10 of all children with autism actually shows some real regression early in life. Another minority appears to deteriorate in adolescence. Nevertheless, in a subgroup of all children with autism, regression is a real and very important phenomenon. In such cases, fluctuation in

language or behaviour often raises the suspicion of epilepsy. Epilepsy or a paroxysmal EEG occasionally may be associated with autistic regression. However, according to one author, epilepsy probably plays a relatively minor, although non-negligible, pathogenetic role in autistic regression (Rapin 1995). Others (Baird et al. 2006) have not found any evidence of a link. A large study of 200 2–4 year olds with autism spectrum disorders showed that 14% had clear indications of regression. There was no clear link with epilepsy in this subgroup, but low IQ, severity of autistic symptoms and degree of impairment were more prominent than in those without regression (Fernell et al. 2010). Nevertheless, a prolonged sleep EEG that includes study of stage III and stage IV sleep is recommended for children without seizures who have regressed or who have fluctuating deficits and for mute and poorly intelligible children who may have verbal auditory agnosia (Tuchman & Rapin 1997). In the medical literature, there is a rare subgroup of children with chronic motor tics who had both autistic regression and seizures, as described by Nass et al. (1998a, b). Seizures consisted of absence or myoclonic patterns, usually resistant to antiepileptic drugs. The patients had a specific pattern of occipital spiking on EEG.

After language has developed and after 2 years of age, a few children may undergo a rapid regression in language, sociability, play and cognition. This has been called childhood disintegrative disorder (Heller syndrome) and is thought by some to be a separate disorder from classic autism. Some of these cases are almost definitely missed instances of the Landau–Kleffner syndrome.

LANDAU–KLEFFNER (ACQUIRED EPILEPTIC APHASIA) SYNDROME AND ELECTRICAL STATUS EPILEPTICUS IN SLOW-WAVE SLEEP

Landau–Kleffner syndrome is an acquired epileptic aphasia or verbal auditory agnosia affecting children between 2 and 6 years of age who already have developed speech. There are usually clinical seizures and bilateral paroxysmal centro-sylvian EEG pattern. In the classic Landau–Kleffner syndrome, aphasia is acquired and other higher cortical functions may not deteriorate. In a variation of the syndrome called epilepsy with continuous spike-waves during slow-wave sleep (CSWS) or electrical status epilepticus in slow-wave sleep (ESES), speech is disturbed in 50% of the cases and intellectual deterioration occurs, with psychiatric symptoms, often reminiscent of autism, developing. This variant is usually diagnosed after age 6 years. According to Hirsch et al. (1990), they are probably variations of a single syndrome. Continuous and pulsed corticosteroids are usually tried in this patient group and may have at least a temporary – sometimes dramatic – beneficial effect. There is also an experimental surgical therapy called subpial intracortical transection (Chez et al. 1998).

Types of seizures

Many patterns of seizures are seen in patients with autism – infantile spasms, atonic seizures, myoclonic seizures, atypical absence, complex partial seizures and generalised tonic-clonic. Most known EEG patterns also are found in this patient group, including ESES. Infantile spasms and complex partial seizures are relatively more common than other seizure types.

INFANTILE SPASMS AND HYPSARRHYTHMIA (WEST SYNDROME)

Infantile spasms begin in early infancy with multiple axial spasms. The EEG changes have a characteristic picture of abundant spikes and polyspikes along with high-voltage slowing. The association of infantile spasms with this EEG picture of 'hypsarrhythmia' has become known as West syndrome, referring to the physician who first described the features in his own son.

After the infantile spasms have subsided, the child is sometimes left with the development of autistic symptoms. There are also a few descriptions suggesting that the autistic symptoms might have been present at the onset of the overt seizure disorder. The percentage of patients with infantile spasms who later show the symptoms of autism varies in different studies from 2% (Prats et al. 1991) to 16% (Riikonen & Amnell 1981). Millichap (1997) estimates that the percentage who meet the criteria for autism averages around 10%. Looking at the problem from a different perspective, one could ask what percentage of patients with autism with all forms of epilepsy have infantile spasms? In the large series of 302 patients with autism studied by Tuchman et al. (1991), infantile spasms occurred in 12% of those patients with autism who also had epilepsy. In a recent study from Iceland, infantile spasms predicted a very high risk for autistic spectrum disorders (ASD) but this was to a large extent explained by the association of ASD with symptomatic origin of seizures (Saemundsen et al. 2008).

Patients with infantile spasms who later develop an autistic syndrome may have one of a number of different disease entities, placing these patients in the category of a child with one of the double syndromes. Those disease entities that may have infantile spasms in early infancy include tuberous sclerosis, neurofibromatosis 1, Down syndrome, phenylketonuria and minor hydrocephalus. Tuberous sclerosis is one of the more common aetiologies underlying autism. In a study of 38 patients with tuberous sclerosis and epilepsy, 17 had infantile spasms (Ohtsuka et al. 1998). A number of patients with neurofibromatosis 1 also have been reported with infantile spasms (Millichap 1997). (For more details on these double syndromes, see Chapter 11.)

One study suggests that both temporal lobes often appear to be involved in those patients with infantile spasms who will later develop autism (Chugani et al. 1996). This follow-up study of 14 infants with infantile spasms and a positron emission tomography (PET) study which showed bitemporal hypometabolism revealed that 10 had developed autism.

In the first few weeks of life, infantile spasm is the seizure pattern most likely, by far, to be associated with later development of autistic symptoms. However, there is a case in the literature of a child with EEG and clinical symptoms that met the criteria of benign familial neonatal convulsions who later developed autism (Alfonso et al. 1997).

ATONIC SEIZURES

Atonic seizures refer to generalised seizures in which the dominant motor manifestation is loss of postural tone, associated with loss of consciousness, usually for several minutes. They are simply generalised motor seizures with limpness, rather than stiffness and repetitive jerking. Such cases have been reported in children with autism in the Tuchman et al. (1991) series.

MYOCLONIC EPILEPSIES OF EARLY CHILDHOOD (MINOR MOTOR SEIZURES)

Myoclonic seizures refer to single or multiple brief, shock-like jerking movements of the head, trunk or extremities. The infant form of these epilepsies begins in infancy or preschool years and often is seen in combination with tonic-clonic patterns. It may be associated with bursts of slow 1–2.5 per second spike-and-wave complexes on EEG.

Myoclonic seizures are seen in patients with autism but it is unusual to find them as an isolated seizure type. Most often, they are found in combination with other seizure patterns, particularly tonic-clonic, and are classified as the myoclonic epilepsies (Gillberg & Steffenburg 1987, Olsson et al. 1988). As the exception to the rule, there are several cases in the medical literature of solitary myoclonic seizures and autism (Boyer et al. 1981, Gillberg 1984). The Gillberg (1984) case is a description of a boy with classic autism and myoclonic seizures who became seizure free on valproic acid and thereafter quickly improved regarding both his severe behavioural symptoms and his language disturbances.

ABSENCE EPILEPSY (PETIT MAL)

Absence seizures refer to staring spells, usually less than 20 seconds in duration, sometimes with slight flickering of the eyes. There are associated bilateral 2–4 Hz spike-and-slow wave complexes on EEG. EEGs are indicated for children in whom epilepsy is suspected, but it should be kept in mind that non-epileptic staring spells are much more common than absence seizures (Rapin 1997).

There are a few studies which have found absence seizures in patients with autism (Ritvo et al. 1990, Tuchman et al. 1991). The absence seizures may be described as atypical. There is a case in the literature of an 8-year-old boy in whom absence seizures were reported to 'masquerade' as autism. He had almost continuous bilateral synchronous 3 Hz spike-and-slow wave on EEG and improved dramatically, both psychiatrically and neurologically, with ethosuximide monotherapy (Gillberg & Schaumann 1983).

COMPLEX PARTIAL SEIZURES (PSYCHOMOTOR EPILEPSY)

If a child blanks out or stares, there are two possible seizure types to consider. One is absence seizures, as described above. The other is complex partial seizures which usually last between 30 seconds and 3 minutes and are accompanied by a variety of automatisms, such as lip smacking, hand wringing or plucking at clothes. Other signs of a partial complex seizure might be a temporary 'dreamy state' or impaired consciousness with an affective disturbance such as fear or anger. The EEG may show either unilateral or bilateral foci, usually frontal or temporal.

It is easy to see how such seizure activity might be hard to pick out in a child with autism. Corbett (1982) raised the question about how likely it was that such seizure activity might be under-reported in non-verbal children with autism. A population-based study of epilepsy in prepubertal children with autism or autistic-like conditions found that complex partial seizures were present in 71% of those who had an onset of seizures in early childhood (Olsson et al. 1988). In another study of young people with autism, aged 16–23 years, Gillberg & Steffenburg (1987) found that the majority of those with epilepsy and a prepubertal onset had complex partial seizures. Danielsson, following children with autism from early chldhood into young-middle adulthood, has since reported that complex partial seizures are the most common type of seizures in autism (Danielsson et al. 2005).

GENERALISED TONIC-CLONIC SEIZURES (GRAND MAL)

In seizure parlance, the word 'tonic' refers to a stiffening of the body with rigid extension of the trunk and extremities. The word 'clonic' refers to generalised seizures with repetitive bilateral clonic jerking of the extremities. In tonic-clonic (grand mal) seizures, there is typically alternate stiffening and jerking associated with loss of consciousness.

Generalised tonic-clonic seizures are the most frequent form of epilepsy in the general population. They are relatively common in children and adolescents with autism (Carod et al. 1995, Olsson et al. 1988, Tuchman et al. 1991). In autism, tonic-clonic seizures may be associated with other types of seizures, either as a sequela after infantile spasms or immediately following complex partial seizures (Gillberg & Steffenburg 1987, Olsson et al. 1988). However, clinical descriptions vary widely in the rigor of enquiry about early features of the seizure and the precise motor phenomena.

Electrophysiology

There are now many papers on the EEG findings in individuals with autism with and without epilepsy. Some of these have been on very large samples and have shown that, using 24-hour ambulatory EEG recordings, epileptiform abnormalities can be identified in sleep in as many as 60% of the whole group (of almost 900 individuals), even in individuals with no recorded overt clinical seizures. The most common locality for such abnormalities has been in the right temporal lobe (Chez et al. 2006).

One of the most difficult things to evaluate in the field of autism is the many papers describing brainstem auditory evoked potentials, cortical evoked potentials and event-related potentials in these patients. The difficulty arises because the studies done by outstanding investigators have been found to contradict each other. The studies are remarkable in their lack of a coherent answer to specific questions. Even studies with large numbers of patients – 109 children in the Wong & Wong (1991) study – are contradicted by other studies (Klin 1993). The inconsistent literature is particularly disappointing because of the greater consistency of results of such studies in developmental syndromes which have more specifically defined aetiologies, such as Down syndrome.

A glimpse of what might help to explain this confusing literature is provided by the electrophysiological studies performed by the Lelord group in France (Lelord et al. 1993, Martineau et al. 1992a, b). Their studies agree that the cognitive deficit in the ability to maintain cross-modal associations is preceded by a more elementary perceptive abnormality in children with autism. What is illuminating is that they interpret their results as allowing the separation of children with autism into three subgroups who presented different patterns of ability to form cross-modal associations. The three subgroups presented different clinical profiles regarding attention, intention, motility, association, contact and communication.

Another possible explanation for the inconsistent results is the chance that calcium levels in the brain of those being studied might vary from patient to patient. A subgroup of children with autism (not negligible in size) have abnormal calcium levels in the urine.

It has been shown in the medical literature on dialysis that the lower the calcium level, the greater the brainstem auditor evoked response (BAER) absolute latency and interpeak latency values (Pratt et al. 1986). Thivièrge et al. (1990), in their BAER study of 20 children with autism, did not attempt to measure calcium levels although they were puzzled by the contradictory results in the literature and came up with the suggestion that calcium levels in the brainstem might help explain the incompatible reports from excellent centres.

Thus, there is a possibility that a population of children with autism, even though they are carefully diagnosed, is not homogeneous regarding many electrophysiological phenomena. When scientists start their experiments with mixed populations, there will be inevitable variability in the results – no matter how carefully a study is performed, how brilliant the investigator or how sophisticated the equipment. In the future, when electrophsyiological studies are performed on specific disease entities within the autistic syndrome, data which will survive the test of time are likely to emerge.

New variations of electrophysiological studies have been introduced into the field but are still based on studying all patients with autism mixed together as one whole. Midlatency auditory evoked responses (P1), measuring the ascending reticular activating system and its thalamic target cells, have been reported as abnormal in children with autism (Buchwald et al. 1992). Studies from The Netherlands have shown that the occipital event-related potential P3 waves are smaller in children with autism compared to controls (Verbaten et al. 1991). In 1994, Kemner et al. compared children with autism with three control groups (normal, attention-deficit, dyslexic) and found that they differed from controls with respect to visual and somatosensory event-related potential P2N2 and the visual event-related potential P3; these authors also found that children with autism show abnormalities of processing of both proximal (somatosensory) and distal (visual) stimuli. The studies raise the question of understimulation of the occipital lobe by visual stimuli in autism (Kemner et al. 1995). A reassuring study, evaluating speech prosody, indicated 'remarkably normal P3 and behavioral processing of prosodic stimuli by high-functioning adults' with autism (Erwin et al. 1991).

One recent theory for the neural basis of autism involves dysfunction in the mirror neurone systems in the brain (Williams 2008). Several lines of evidence, including EEG findings of abnormal mu-rhythms (Stroganova et al. 2007, Oberman et al. 2008), indicate that such dysfunction is indeed much more common in autism than in comparison groups, although the specificity of the findings (for autism) remains to be established. A Swedish–Russian EEG collaboration project has also shown imbalance in the excitatory/inhibitory systems in the brain, with ineffective inhibitory control of sensory processing (Orekhova et al. 2008).

Conclusion

Individuals with an autistic syndrome are more likely to have a seizure disorder than most categories of individuals with intellectual disability. There are data to suggest that even in the absence of intellectual disability, epilepsy is much over-represented in autism spectrum disorders. Conversely, people who suffer seizure disorders are at hugely increased risk of also having autistic features. Some disease entities within the autistic syndrome include patients with epilepsy; others do not. Some types of epilepsy are more likely to be associated with epilepsy – including infantile spasms, complex partial seizures, and the Landau–Kleffner and ESES syndromes.

It is likely that the association seen between autism and epilepsy (and vice versa) represents a conglomerate of findings: coincidence, comorbidity, underlying brain pathology leading to both types of problem, and epileptogenic activity (and antiepileptic drug treatment) causing autistic behaviour in some cases.

Whether or not epilepsy and autism should be regarded as comorbid, coexisting, associated with an underlying common brain abnormality or related by way of one condition leading to the other is a contentious issue and there are examples of cases in which it would be appropriate to consider each of these options. There are probably coincidentally comorbid – very rare – cases of autism and epilepsy, many others where the coexistence is non-coincidental but the reason for the coexistence remains obscure, yet others (such as in tuberous sclerosis) where both epilepsy and autism are caused by the same underlying brain disorder, and others still where the epileptic activity *per se* leads on to autistic symptomatology (such as in some cases of Landau–Kleffner syndrome and other more unspecified epileptic encephalopathies).

The case described by Humphrey et al. (2006) is of particular interest in relation to the possible role of the epileptic seizures *per se* in the generation of autistic symptoms. An infant was diagnosed as having tuberous sclerosis at age 6 months. He was put on vigabatrin because of epileptogenic discharge on the EEG and seizures but the medication was discontinued 7 months later. He was developing normally and had no autistic features at 12 and 18 months. However, seizures recurred at age 21 months and on evaluation at 24 months he did meet criteria for autism and intellectual disability.

There are probably also cases where treatment of epileptogenic discharge on the EEG can itself lead to resolution of autistic symptomatology (Gillberg & Schauman 1983), and yet other instances in which antiepileptic treatment can lead to marked autistic features in individuals who did not have such features before starting treatment and who improved dramatically when taken off the drug (in the experience of the author, some of the benzodiazepines have this potential).

Finally, epilepsy and autism can be linked in a very different way, through maternal epilepsy in pregnancy increasing the risk that the child may later show epilepsy and autism for genetic reasons, but also as a consequence of antiepileptic treatment with, for example, valproic acid (Bryant & Dreifuss 1996).

In any case, all individuals with the combination of autism and epilepsy need to be worked up on the basis of understanding that there is not one cause explaining the link between the two. Individual diagnosis and treatment is the best approach to epilepsy in autism, and to autism in epilepsy.

NOTE

This is an updated version of a chapter originally published in *The Biology of the Autistic Syndromes,* edited by C. Gillberg and M. Coleman, Mac Keith Press, London, 2000.

REFERENCES

Alfonso I, Hahn JS, Papazian O, Martinez YL, Reyes MA, Aicardi J (1997) Bilateral tonic-clonic epileptic seizures in non-benign familial neonatal convulsions. *Pediatr Neurol* **16**, 249–251.

Amiet C, Gourfinkel-An I, Bouzamondo A, et al. (2008) Epilepsy in autism is associated with intellectual disability and gender: evidence from a meta-analysis. *Biol Psychiatry* **64**, 577–582.

Baird G, Robinson RO, Boyd S, Charman T. (2006) Sleep electroencephalograms in young children with autism with and without regression. *Dev Med Child Neurol* **48**, 604–608.

Billstedt E, Gillberg IC, Gillberg C (2005) Autism after adolescence: population-based 13–22-year follow-up study of 120 individuals with autism diagnosed in childhood. *J Autism Dev Disord* **35**, 351–360.

Billstedt E, Gillberg IC, Gillberg C (2007) Autism in adults: symptoms patterns and early childhood predictors. Use of the DISCO in a community sample followed from childhood. *J Child Psychol Psychiatry* **48**, 1102–1110.

Boyer J-P, Deschatrette A, Delwarde M (1981) Autism convulsif? (in French) *Pédiatrie* **5**, 353–368.

Bryant AE III, Dreifuss FE (1996) Valproic hepatic fatalities. III. US experience since 1986. *Neurology* **46**, 465–469.

Buchwald JS, Erwin R, van Lancker D, Guthrie D, Schwafel J, Tanguay P (1992) Midlatency auditory evoked responses: P1 abnormalities in adult autistic subjects. *Electroencephalograph Clin Neurophysiol* **84**, 164–171.

Carod FJ, Prats JM, Garaizar C, Zuazo E (1995) Clinical-radiological evaluation of infantile autism and epileptic syndromes associated with autism. (in Spanish) *Rev Neurol* **23**, 1203–1207.

Cederlund M, Hagberg B, Billstedt E, Gillberg IC, Gillberg C (2008) Asperger syndrome and autism – a comparative longitudinal follow-up study more than 5 years after original diagnosis. *J Autism Dev Disord* **38**, 72–85.

Chez MG, Loeffel M, Buchanan CP, Field-Chez M (1998) Pulse high-dose steroids as combination therapy with valproic acid in epileptic aphasia patients with pervasive developmental delay or autism. *Ann Neurol* **44**, 539.

Chez MG, Chang M, Krasne V, Coughlan C, Kominsky M, Schwartz A (2006) Frequency of epileptiform EEG abnormalities in a sequential screening of autistic patients with no known clinical epilepsy from 1996 to 2005. *Epilepsy Behav* **8**, 267–271.

Chugani HT, da Silva E, Chugani DC (1996) Prognostic implications of bitemporal hypometabolism on positron emission tomography. *Ann Neurol* **39**, 643–649.

Corbett J (1982) Epilepsy and the electroencephalogram in early childhood psychosis. In: Wing JK, Wing L (eds) *Handbook of Psychiatry*, vol 3. London: Cambridge University Press, pp. 198–202.

Danielsson S, Gillberg IC, Billstedt E, Gillberg C, Olsson I (2005) Epilepsy in young adults with autism: a prospective population-based follow-up study of 120 individuals diagnosed in childhood. *Epilepsia* **46**, 918–923.

Danielsson S, Viggedal G, Steffenburg S, Rydenhag B, Gillberg C, Olsson I (2008) Psychopathology, psychosocial functioning, and IQ before and after epilepsy surgery in children with drug-resistant epilepsy. *Epilepsy Behav* **14**, 330–337.

Elia M, Musumeci SA, Ferri R, Bergonzi P (1995) Clinical and neurophysiological aspects of epilepsy in subjects with autism and mental retardation. *Am J Mental Retard* **100**, 6–16.

Erwin R, van Lancker D, Guthrie D, Schwafel J, Tanguay P, Buchwald JS (1991) P3 responses to prosodic stimuli in adult autistic subject. *Electroencephalograph Clin Neurophysiol* **80**, 561–571.

Fernell E, Hedvall A, Norrelgen F, et al. (2010) Developmental profiles in preschool children with autism spectrum disorders referred for intervention. *Res Dev Disabil* **31**(3), 790–799.

Gillberg C (1984) Infantile autism and other childhood psychoses in a Swedish urban region. Epidemiological aspects. *J Child Psychol Psychiat* **25**, 35–43.

Gillberg C, Schaumann H (1983) Epilepsy presenting as infantile autism? Two case studies. *Neuropediatrics* **14**, 206–212.

Gillberg C, Steffenburg S (1987) Outcome and prognostic factors in infantile autism and similar conditions: a population-based study of 46 cases followed through puberty. *J Autism Dev Disord* **17**, 273–287.

Gillberg C, Persson E, Grufman M, Themnér U (1986) Psychiatric disorders in mildly and severely mentally retarded urban children and adolescents: epidemiological aspects. *Br J Psychiatr* **149**, 68–74.

Herder GA (1993) Infantile autism among children in the county of Nordland. Prevalence and etiology. (in Norwegian) *Tidsskr Nor Laegeforen* **113**, 2247–2249.

Hirsch E, Marescaux C, Maquet P, et al. (1990) Landau–Kleffner syndrome: a clinical and EEG study. *Epilepsia* **31**, 756–767.

Humphrey A, Neville BG, Clarke A, Bolton PF (2006) Autistic regression associated with seizure onset in an infant with tuberous sclerosis. *Dev Med Child Neurol* **48**, 609–611.

Kanner L (1943) Autistic disturbances of affective contact. *Nerv Child* **2**, 217–250.

Kanner L (1971) Follow-up study of eleven children originally reported in 1943. *J Autism Child Schizophren* **1**, 119–145.

Kemner C, Verbaten MC, Cuperus JM, Camfferman G, van Engeland H (1994) Visual and somatosensory event-related brain potentials in autistic children and three different control groups. *Electroencephalograph Clin Neurophysiol* **92**, 225–237.

Kemner C, Verbaten MN, Cuperus JM, Camfferman G, van Engeland H (1995) Auditory event-related brain potentials in autistic children and three different control groups. *Biol Psychiatry* **38**,150–165.

Klin A (1993) Auditory brainstem responses in autism: brainstem dysfunction or peripheral hearing loss? *J Autism Dev Disord* **23**, 15–35.

Lelord G, Herault J, Perrot A, et al. (1993) Childhood autism: a relating deficiency due to a developmental disorder of the nervous system. (in French) *Bull Acad Natl Med* **177**, 1423–1430.

Martineau J, Roux S, Adrien JL, Garreau B, Barthelemy C, Lelord G (1992a) Electrophysiological evidence of different abilities to form cross-modal associations in children with autistic behavior. *Electroencephalogr Clin Neurophysiol* **82**, 60–66.

Martineau J, Roux S, Garreau B, Adrien JL, Lelord G (1992b) Unimodal and crossmodal reactivity in autism: presence of auditory evoked responses and effect of the repetition of auditory stimuli. *Biol Psychiatry* **31**,1190–11203.

Millichap JG (1997) *Progress in Pediatric Neurology III*. Chicago: PNB Publishers, p.41.

Nass R, Gross A, Devinsky O (1998a) Autism and autistic epileptiform regression with occipital spikes. *Dev Med Child Neurol* **40**, 453–458.

Nass R, Gross A, Wisoff J, Devinsky O (1998b) Autistic epileptiform regression: response to multiple subpial resections. *Ann Neurol* **44**, 554.

Oberman LM, Ramachandran VS (2008) Preliminary evidence for deficits in multisensory integration in autism spectrum disorders: the mirror neuron hypothesis. *Soc Neurosci* **3**, 348–355.

Ohtsuka Y, Ohmori I, Oka E (1998) Long-term follow-up of childhood epilepsy associated with tuberous sclerosis. *Epilepsia* **39**, 1158–1163.

Olsson I, Steffenburg S, Gillberg C (1988) Epilepsy in autism and autistic-like conditions: a population-based study. *Arch Neurol* **45**, 666–668.

Orekhova EV, Stroganova TA, Prokofyev AO, Nygren G, Gillberg C, Elam M (2008) Sensory gating in young children with autism: relation to age, IQ, and EEG gamma oscillations. *Neurosci Lett* **434**, 218–223.

Prats JM, Garaizar C, Rua MJ, Garcia-Nieto ML, Madoz P (1991) Infantile spasms treated with high doses of sodium valproate: initial response and follow-up. *Dev Med Child Neurol* **33**, 617–625.

Pratt H, Brosky G, Goldsher M, et al. (1986) Auditory brain stem evoked potentials in patients undergoing dialysis. *Electroencephalograph Clin Neurophysiol* **63**, 18–24.

Rapin I (1995) Autistic regression and disintegrative disorder: how important is the role of epilepsy? *Semin Pediatr Neurol* **2**, 278–285.

Rapin I (1997) Autism. *N Engl J Med* **337**, 97–104.

Riikonen R, Amnell G (1981) Psychiatric disorders in children with earlier infantile spasms. *Dev Med Child Neurol* **23**, 747–760.

Ritvo ER, Freeman BJ, Pingree C, et al. (1990) The UCLA-University of Utah epidemiological survey of autism prevalence. *Am J Psychiatr* **146**, 194–199.

Rossi PG, Parmeggiani A, Bach V, Santucci M, Visconti P (1995) EEG features and epilepsy in patients with autism. *Brain Dev* **17**, 169–174.

Saemundsen E, Ludvigsson P, Rafnsson V (2008) Risk of autism spectrum disorders after infantile spasms: a population-based study nested in a cohort with seizures in the first year of life. *Epilepsia* **49**, 1865–1870.

Steffenburg U, Hagberg G, Viggedal G, Kyllerman M (1995) Active epilepsy in mentally retarded children. I. Prevalence and additional neuro-impairments. *Acta Paediatr* **84**, 1147–1152.

Steffenburg S, Gillberg C, Steffenburg U (1996) Psychiatric disorders in children and adolescents with mental retardation and active epilepsy. *Arch Neurol* **53**, 904–912.

Stroganova TA, Nygren G, Tsetlin MM, et al. (2007) Abnormal EEG lateralization in boys with autism. *Clin Neurophysiol* **118**, 1842–1854.

Thivièrge J, Bedard C, Côté R, Maziade M (1990) Brainstem auditory evoked response and subcortical abnormalities in autism. *Am J Psychiatr* **147**, 1609–1613.

Tsai LY, Tsai MC, August GJ (1985) Brief report: implication of EEG diagnosis in the subclassification of infantile autism. *J Autism Child Schizophren* **15**, 339–344.

Tuchman RF, Rapin I (1997) Regression in pervasive developmental disorders: seizures and epileptiform electroencephalogram correlates. *Pediatrics* **99**, 560–565.

Tuchman RF, Rapin I, Shinnar S (1991) Autistic and dysphasic children. II: epilepsy. *Pediatrics* **88**, 1219–1225.

Verbaten MN, Roelofs JW, van Engeland H, Kenemans JK, Slagen JL (1991) Abnormal visual event-related potentials of autistic children. *J Autism Dev Disord* **21**, 449–470.

Williams JH (2008) Self-other relations in social development and autism: multiple roles for mirror neurons and other brain bases. *Autism Res* **1**, 73–90.

Wong V (1993) Epilepsy in children with autistic spectrum disorder. *J Child Neurol* **8**, 316–322.

Wong V, Wong SN (1991) Brainstem auditory evoked potential study in children with autistic disorder. *J Autism Dev Disord* **23**, 15–35.

7
GENETIC CORRELATES OF PSYCHIATRIC COMORBIDITY: FRAGILE X SYNDROME

Sufen Chiu, David Hessl, Josh Day and Randi Hagerman

Fragile X syndrome (FXS) is the most common known inherited cause of intellectual disability. Although Down syndrome is more common, it is usually sporadic and not inherited from generation to generation affecting multiple members in a family (frequency of Down syndrome is 1/1000 relative to FXS 1/4000). Unlike trisomy 21, however, the genetic defect and phenotypic features of FXS have been less obvious to both the clinician and the research scientist for several reasons. Dr Turner described FXS as an X-linked mental retardation syndrome with macro-orchidism (Turner et al. 1975). Many of the classic features of FXS emerge in childhood after birth, such as the elongated, narrow face and large, prominent ears (Hagerman 2002), making a definitive diagnosis at birth difficult without genetic testing.

Dr Lubs first reported the X-linked mental retardation syndrome when he identified a 'marker X chromosome' in 1969. In addition, Dr Cliff Judge, a psychiatrist and geneticist in Australia, clinically described some of the first cases of FXS. As recognition of this syndrome developed, other characteristic features were described that included velvet-like skin, hyperextensible finger joints, high arched palate, flat feet, pectus excavatum and mitral valve prolapse. These features are considered part of the phenotype rather than comorbidities because of the presence of elastin abnormalities (Hagerman 2002).

Molecular biology of fragile X syndrome

In 1991, several laboratories independently identified the area of genetic vulnerability on the X chromosome as containing excessive repeats of a specific, short DNA sequence, a trinucleotide repeat $(CGG)_n$ (Kremer et al. 1991, Verkerk et al. 1991, Vincent et al. 1991, Bell et al. 1991, Hagerman 2002). The expanded CGG repeat results in excessive methylation of the fragile X mental retardation 1 gene (FMR1). Methylation is now recognised as a process for shutting genes down so that they do not get transcribed into mRNA (Kremer et al. 1991, Verkerk et al. 1991, Jin et al. 2002). Therefore, the protein encoded by the DNA in that region is absent because there is no mRNA to translate.

The trinucleotide DNA sequence, CGG, is repeated from 200 to over 2000 times near the promoter region of the FMR1 gene on the X chromosome in individuals with FXS (Brown 2002, Fu et al. 1991). A premutation carrier state found in individuals who transmit the mutation to their offspring is defined as having between 55 and 200 repeats of CGG.

The offspring of female carriers will often expand to >2000 CGG repeats, the full mutation resulting in FXS.

This phenomenon of expansion of DNA across generations is a novel, disease-causing genetic mechanism that was unknown prior to the discovery of this mutation in FXS (Cummings & Zoghbi 2000). It helps to explain 'anticipation' which describes the phenomenon of a disorder that increases in frequency and/or severity and presents at earlier ages with succeeding generations in a family. Anticipation is now proposed to explain a wide variety of disorders including psychiatric illnesses such as autism, bipolar disorder and schizophrenia (Ross et al. 1993, Carpenter 1994, O'Donovan et al. 1995, Petronis & Kennedy 1995, Ashworth et al. 1996, Margolis et al. 1997, Vincent et al. 2000). Therefore, this novel genetic model of disease, anticipation, may result from the 'instability' of the DNA giving rise to the expansion of the same trinucleotide repeat in successive generations, ultimately resulting in illness in more family members with increasing severity at a younger age. To date, the majority of these disorders are autosomal dominant or X-linked (Cummings & Zoghbi 2000).

A minority of individuals who have the full mutation have some proportion of cells in the body that contain less than 200 repeats and function normally (Rousseau 1994). These individuals traditionally are called 'mosaics'. Alternatively, some individuals demonstrate 'methylation mosaicism' where all of their cells have the full mutation but only partial methylation results and some protein translation occurs (Nolin et al. 1994).

Several lines of research have demonstrated that the FMR1 protein binds specific messenger mRNAs and regulates the translation of these RNAs into proteins (Brown et al. 2001, O'Donnell & Warren 2002). In addition, other evidence suggests that the FMR1 mRNA may play a regulatory role in the cells, known as RNA interference (Siomi et al. 2004). RNA interference is a post-transcriptional process by which RNAs are specifically silenced or destroyed by other RNAs.

Another novel genetic mechanism that results in disease has been revealed by studies regarding the type and amount of mRNA produced by the FMR1 gene that can modify cellular processes (Hagerman & Hagerman 2004). The CGG in the promoter region of the FMR1 gene does not alter the structure of FMRP but modulates when and how much FMRP to make from the FMR1 mRNA template of the gene. In premutation individuals, the increased number of CGG repeats within the premutation range does not limit the transcription of the gene into RNA. On the contrary, the FMR1 mRNA levels are elevated in individuals with the premutation (Tassone et al. 2000a). The extra repeats contained in the RNA promoter region interfere with the translation process, leading often to a mild deficiency of FMRP (Chen et al. 2003).

The identification of the genetic mutation in FXS has engendered several new genetic models for disease. DNA expansion helps to explain the phenomenon of anticipation, where certain disorders appear to increase in frequency, with increased severity, at younger ages in successive generations of affected families. The absence of FMRP in FXS interferes with the translation of many mRNAs that involve multiple systems, resulting in the complex pattern of morbidity associated with this disorder.

Comorbidities of fragile X syndrome

Even though the molecular biology of FXS syndrome has been carefully studied, it remains a devastating disorder with significant comorbidities (Hagerman & Hagerman 2002). The identification of the DNA abnormality associated with FXS has clarified its unique transmission pattern, developmental heterogeneity and varied phenotypic expression. Therefore, the genetic mechanisms identified to date provide a clearer explanation as to which of these comorbidities is actually a part of a broader phenotype.

Intellectual disability

Traditionally, intellectual disability of moderate to severe degree represents the cardinal feature of FXS and other genetic syndromes associated with intellectual disability. Often when the degree of intellectual impairment is absent, genetic syndromes are not considered in the differential diagnosis of behavioural problems. Accumulating clinical experience along with definitive diagnoses via genetic testing are proving that the spectrum of intellectual disability in FXS is broader than ever imagined, ranging from severe intellectual disability and autism to specific learning disorders with relatively intact overall intellectual ability. The genetic model that may explain this range of phenotypic expression in cognitive disability has evolved from the identification of full mutation individuals who have partial methylation or complete lack of methylation of the FMR1 gene. Unlike the full mutation individuals with complete methylation, these individuals have a level of FMRP that correlates with their intellectual ability (Tassone et al. 1999, Loesch et al. 2004).

One of the specific learning disabilities associated with FXS includes problems with arithmetic reasoning and digit span as measured by cognitive testing (Kemper et al. 1986, Brainard et al. 1991, Rivera et al. 2002). This arithmetic disability may be similar to that seen in other genetic syndromes including Turner syndrome and velocardiofacial syndrome (Simon et al. 2005). In FXS, the degree of impairment in arithmetic ability appears to correlate with the amount of FMRP (Rivera et al. 2002). This arithmetic disability is distinct from problems with attention also found in FXS.

Attention problems in FXS are attributed to a deficit in executive function above and beyond that found in comparable developmentally delayed children and cognitively matched, typically developing children with attention-deficit–hyperactivity disorder (ADHD) (Munir et al. 2000). The most notable difference is that individuals with FXS more often perseverate on previous correct responses because of an inability to switch visual attention and inhibit repetitive behaviour (Wilding et al. 2002). Therefore, attentional problems associated with executive function are more impaired in FXS than the level of cognitive function would predict.

Vocabulary and syntactic language appears to be spared in FXS but greater deficits occur in conversational language ability that manifests itself as tangential, perseverative, repetitive and echolalic speech (Cornish et al. 2004). Increased frequency of these errors is postulated to correlate with heightened arousal during social interactions even though face and emotion recognition is intact. Therefore, specific language impairments, attentional difficulties and maths disability represent a specific cognitive deficit profile occurring in FXS in addition to global intellectual disability.

Psychosis and fragile X syndrome

Individuals with intellectual disability suffer more often from comorbid psychiatric disorders. General estimates are as high as 40% (Einfeld & Tonge 1996, Hardan & Sahl 1997). However, screening tools for psychiatric disorders are limited and thought to often overestimate the prevalence of psychopathology. Given the social difficulties associated with intellectual disability, higher rates of psychiatric disorder are to be expected. Nevertheless, certain psychiatric disorders, such as anxiety and psychotic disorders, may be over-represented in FXS. The obsessive-compulsive disorder is part of the clinical picture of a Prader–Willi sub-phenotype of FXS that also includes hypogenitalia (Hagerman & Hagerman 2002). The evidence for how anxiety and psychotic disorders may be subphenotypes of FXS rather than comorbidities is examined in depth here.

Psychosis is a disabling condition that often presents as a comorbid condition in individuals with intellectual disability. Estimates of psychosis in the intellectual disabled population suggest rates as high as 10% (Hardan & Sahl 1997, Prosser et al. 1998, Benassi et al. 1990). New molecular evidence suggests that individuals with FXS may be even more vulnerable to psychosis. A recent study by Antar and colleagues showed that the metabotropic glutamate receptor (mGluR5) regulates the localisation and trafficking of FMRP and FMR1 mRNA to dendrites and synapses (Antar et al. 2004). An earlier study suggested that the group 1 metabotropic glutamate receptor activation was required for FMRP-mediated translation of PSD-95, a scaffolding protein important to synaptic plasticity (Todd et al. 2003). Another theory suggests that the group 1 metabotropic glutamate receptor activation (Gp 1 mGluR) promotes protein synthesis-dependent long-term depression (LTD) (Bear et al. 2004). LTD is exaggerated in FMRP-deficient mice. FMRP synthesis is induced by Gp 1 mGLu R activation and therefore FMRP may be important in dampening LTD in a feedback loop. The net effect of exaggerated LTD is slowing of synaptic maturation that results in intellectual disability and perhaps psychosis.

Schizophrenia has been postulated to be a disorder of the synapse given the lack of significant gross structural abnormalities of the brain (Harrison & Weinberger 2004). Alterations in glutamate neurotransmission in the hippocampus and cerebellum have been associated with schizophrenia. These areas of the brain, the hippocampus and cerebellum, are also thought to play a role in the pathophysiology of FXS (Hessl et al. 2004a). The complex interaction of glutamate and dopamine, the classic neurotransmitter associated with schizophrenia, is currently being elaborated (Harrison & Weinberger 2004). For example, dopamine is required for or facilitates LTD that results from Gp1 mGluR activation (Otani et al. 2003).

These observations may also explain neuroanatomical changes common to schizophrenia and FXS. In both disorders, increased lateral ventricular volume has been reported (Guerreiro et al. 1998, Humra et al. 2000, Eliez et al. 2001). A decrease in the medial-temporal lobe volumes was found in adult schizophrenia studies (McCarley et al. 1999) but not reproduced in studies of childhood-onset schizophrenia (COS). Kumra and colleagues (2000) proposed that abnormalities in the medial-temporal lobe might develop later in adolescence. In FXS, a decrease in temporal lobe volume has been reported (Reiss et al. 1994).

Another deficit common to schizophrenia and FXS is an alteration in prepulse inhibition (PPI), observed clinically as the inability to suppress motor response to irrelevant environmental stimuli (Le Pen & Moreau 2002, Frankland et al. 2004). Le Pen and colleagues show that the alterations in PPI are reversible with the new atypical antipsychotics but not by a typical antipsychotic, haloperidol. Interestingly, Frankland and colleagues showed a correlation between the degree of PPI alteration and severity of autistic symptoms in FXS. Abnormalities in PPI in autism spectrum disorders without FXS are also beginning to be identified (McAlonan et al. 2002). Therefore, the increased use of atypical antipsychotic medications in treating the symptoms of autism and FXS in addition to schizophrenia may be related to reversing deficits in PPI (McCracken et al. 2002, Berry-Kravis & Potanos 2004).

Schizophrenia is one of the most devastating psychiatric disorders and much research has shed little light on its genetic causes (Tsuang et al. 2000). Prior to the discovery of the FXS genetic models of disease, previous genetic theories were inadequate to explain a disease that most often presented during adolescence through early adulthood without obvious signs of disease or pathological process in the brain. If the FXS mutation is associated with psychosis, which is in the same spectrum of schizophrenia, RNA binding studies with FMRP may identify the group of genes that contribute to the development of schizophrenia. Methylation mosaicism, leading to a double hit of lowered FMRP and elevated FMR1 mRNA, may also explain some forms of schizophrenia.

Anxiety and fragile X syndrome

These same molecular pathways may play a role in the over-representation of anxiety disorders in FXS. The anxiety disorders of FXS span social anxiety, general anxiety and obsessive-compulsive disorder. Early childhood studies of FXS suggest that these anxiety traits are present well before the chronicity of illness starts to take its toll.

Anxiety is one of the most prominent behavioural features of FXS. The anxiety is typically manifested by avoidance of eye contact, especially in novel social situations. Other behaviours seem to co-occur with anxiety and hyperarousal, such as increased aggression, tangential speech and cluttering, and stereotypic behaviours, but these observations have not been substantiated in empirical studies. Other symptoms of anxiety, such as physiological arousal, subjective experiences of nervousness and panic, have been difficult to evaluate in this population due to limitations in insight and expressive language level. The anxiety and accompanying behaviours observed in individuals with FXS may be associated with autism in this population. These individuals may avert their gaze, due to overstimulation and social anxiety, demonstrate stereotypical behaviours and be diagnosed with autism despite having a strong interest in relating to others and otherwise developmentally appropriate social reciprocity. The severity of internalising types of behaviour problems is correlated with the FMRP deficit in children with FXS, even after accounting for a number of other factors such as background predisposition to psychopathology in parents and features of the home environment, suggesting a more direct impact of the FMR1 gene dysfunction of these types of behaviours (Hessl et al. 2001).

Psychophysiology studies document that individuals with FXS respond with heightened physiological responses to sensory and social stimuli. Children with fragile X have increased galvanic skin responses to visual, auditory, tactile, vestibular and olfactory stimuli (Miller et al. 1999), reflecting abnormal activation of the sympathetic nervous system. In comparison to developmental matched peers, they also have increased galvanic skin responses when first meeting an unfamiliar adult (Hessl et al. 2004b). In conjunction with the enhanced sympathetic response, individuals with fragile X also have reduced vagal tone, a measure of parasympathetic influence on the heart associated with emotion regulation (Roberts et al. 2001). Hessl and colleagues (2002) measured hypothalamic-pituitary-adrenal (HPA) axis function via sampling of salivary cortisol in a matched sample of 109 children with the fragile X full mutation and 109 of their unaffected siblings. They found that children with FXS, especially males, had significantly higher levels of cortisol during both in-home evaluation (most notably during cognitive and social challenge) and on two typical weekend days (basal cortisol). In addition, elevations in cortisol were significantly associated with the severity of behaviour problems in both boys and girls with FXS, even after accounting for other factors associated with behaviour such as FMRP and IQ.

In addition to cognitive impairment, individuals with FXS often experience high levels of behavioural distress and anxiety, gaze avoidance and withdrawn behaviour, especially when confronted with novel social situations. These problems often lead to major disruptions in daily life and children typically become increasingly socially avoidant and withdrawn over time. Lachiewicz (1992) found that 47% of girls with FXS had scores on the Child Behavior Checklist (CBCL) of greater than the 98th centile for social withdrawal and hyperactivity. Freund and colleagues (1993) furthered this research by carrying out psychiatric evaluations on 17 females with FXS ranging in age from 4 to 27 years. They found a diagnosis of avoidant personality disorder (a rather severe form of shyness and social anxiety) in 65% compared to 12% of IQ- and age-matched controls. Furthermore, Lachiewicz & Dawson (1994) found that 40% of girls with FXS over 9 years of age had an anxiety rating that included shy and fearful behaviour in the clinical range, compared to none of the comparison individuals. More recently, in a large representative in-home study, 42% of boys and 40% of girls with FXS had CBCL social problem scores above the 98th centile, in comparison to just 7% of their unaffected biological siblings (Hessl et al. 2001).

Autism and fragile X syndrome
A higher than expected occurrence of autism appears to affect individuals with FXS. Estimates range from 25% to 30% of individuals with FXS (Bailey et al. 1998, Rogers et al. 2001). Some argue that this is simply a comorbidity of the intellectual disability that occurs in FXS whereas others have proposed a double-hit theory of having two genetic vulnerabilities (Feinstein & Reiss 1998). Rogers and colleagues (2001) screened individuals with FXS for autism with the Autism Diagnostic Observations Schedule (ADOS) and Autism Diagnostic Interview Revised (ADI-R). To address the inherent inability of either diagnostic scale to separate severe intellectual disability from autism, they compared FXS to similarly developmentally disabled individuals with and without autism. Those who had FXS with autism were most similar to individuals with developmental disorders and autism. Individu-

als with FXS only were similar to those with developmental disorders without autism. Therefore, autism is now thought to be over-represented in FXS and not simply a comorbidity of low intellectual function.

Other lines of evidence suggest that many similarities exist between FXS and autism. The possibility of autism being part of the phenotype of FXS was first suggested by Brown and colleagues (1982). Imaging studies of the brain in FXS and autism show that both conditions present with above average brain size and smaller cerebellar size. Typically, most disorders associated with intellectual disabilities have smaller total brain size. As described earlier, there may also be similar deficits in PPI that are reversed by antipsychotic medications. Autism has also been proposed to be a disorder of the synapse because of the lack of gross structural abnormalities (Akshoomoff et al. 2002). Some of these alterations may be related to allelic variations in glutamatergic transporter and receptor genes that have been shown to have linkage disequilibrium in autism (Jamain et al. 2002, Muhle et al. 2004, Serajee et al. 2003) and specifically in the cerebellum (Purcell et al. 2001).

As described earlier, an alteration in PPI is observed clinically as hypersensitivity to environmental stimuli in individuals with FXS with a correlation between the degree of PPI alteration and severity of autistic symptoms (Le Pen & Moreau 2002, Frankland et al. 2004). The abnormalities in PPI in autism (McAlonan et al. 2002) may stem from defects in the limbic system. A major brain region that regulates the limbic system is the amygdala (Amaral et al. 2003).

Amaral and colleagues reported significant differences in the development of the amygdala in children with autism compared to typically developing controls (Schumann et al. 2004). Children with autism have a larger amygdala volume. These differences disappear in adolescence. Similar findings may be present in children with FXS (Hessl et al. 2004a).

Alterations in the HPA axis may also give rise to similar deficits in the limbic system in autism and FXS (Hessl et al. 2002, 2004a). Cortisol is routinely measured to access the role of the HPA axis in psychiatric pathology. In children with FXS, increased cortisol levels were associated with more behavioural problems. Investigators have also reported hypersecretion of cortisol in children with autism (Richdale & Prior 1992, Jansen et al. 2003).

Differences exist in autism compared to FXS, which are highlighted by functional magnetic resonance imaging (fMRI) studies. Using the blood oxygenated level dependence (BOLD) response, which is a measure of blood flow to areas of the brain during specific tasks, fMRI may provide clues as to which areas of the brain may not be functioning in behavioural problems rather than relying on changes in the size of these regions. Reiss and colleagues used fMRI to demonstrate that gaze aversion in FXS was not associated with increase activation of the amygdala, which would have occurred in hyperaroused states associated with anxiety (Garrett et al. 2004). This study demonstrated equal activation of the fusiform gyrus (FG) in individuals with FXS to forward-facing and angled faces. In the controls there was preferential activation of the FG to forward-facing faces. In contrast, greater FG activation occurs in autism than in controls in response to familiar faces compared to faces of strangers (Pierce et al. 2004). However, no studies have carefully evaluated these tasks to determine if they differentiate autism alone from FXS with autism and FXS without autism.

Many neuroanatomical and neurophysiological similarities exist between autism and FXS. Clearly, those with both conditions appear to have a second hit as originally proposed by Feinstein and colleagues. Individuals with FXS and autism have a lower IQ (Bailey et al. 2001, Rogers et al. 2001), worse receptive language (Philofsky et al. 2004), lower adaptive skills and lower social ability (Rogers et al. 2001). Other currently unidentified gene expressions modulated epistatically through FMRP may be responsible for this additive effect, which creates autism in such a large number of individuals with FXS.

The premutation and fragile X-associated tremor/ataxia syndrome
Clinical involvement was first considered in patients with the premutation when the problems appeared to be a mild version of the fragile X behavioural or cognitive phenotype, including anxiety, social avoidance or shyness, learning difficulites with rare intellectual disability or autism (Hagerman et al. 1996, Sobesky et al. 1996, Riddle et al. 1998, Tassone et al. 2000a, Aziz et al. 2003). When measures of FMRP became available, a mild deficit of FMRP became evident that could explain the involvement in most of the affected premutation carriers (Hagerman et al. 1996, Tassone et al. 2000a, Goodlin-Jones et al. 2004). More importantly, clinical manifestations specific to individuals with the premutation and not present in full mutation carriers appear to exist. Only individuals with the premutation were more likely to have premature ovarian failure, occurring in about 20% of women with the premutation (Allingham-Hawkins et al. 1999).

The finding by Tassone et al. (2000b) of elevated FMR1-mRNA in carriers of the premutation confirmed that there was a molecular abnormality in these carriers which did not occur in those with a full mutation. The elevation of the mRNA may be a secondary translation defect in converting the mRNA into FMRP. The excess CGG repeats present in the mRNA interfere in the translation process (Otani et al. 2003, Hagerman & Hagerman 2004, Pietrobono et al. 2005). Although the majority of individuals with the premutation have FMRP levels in the normal range, which typically is associated with a normal or higher IQ (Loesch et al. 2004), some have intellectual disability or autism associated with abnormal levels of FMRP (Tassone et al. 2000a, Aziz et al. 2003, Goodlin-Jones et al. 2004).

Coincident with the documentation of elevated mRNA in carriers, a number of carrier grandfathers were experiencing tremor and ataxia in later life. They all appear to have a similar neurological phenotype (Hagerman et al. 2001), which was named for this constellation of neurological symptoms as the fragile X-associated tremor/ataxia syndrome or FXTAS (Jacquemont et al. 2004). It can begin with either an intention tremor or ataxia. It also includes a peripheral neuropathy with decreased pinprick and vibration sense in the distal lower extremities, memory and executive function deficits, anxiety and mood lability. On MRI, the brain had atrophy and white matter disease particularly involving the middle cerebellar peduncles (Brunberg et al. 2002, Jacquemont et al. 2003).

The neuropathology associated with FXTAS involves the formation of eosinophilic intranuclear inclusions that are τ and α-synuclean negative (Greco et al. 2002). These inclusions occur in the neurones and astrocytes, most abundant in the hippocampus, but are seen throughout the cortex and the cerebellum. Interestingly, they are not present in Purkinje cells. The inclusions contain FMR1- mRNA and other proteins which are important for neuronal function (Hagerman & Hagerman 2004). The excess FMR1 mRNA in the premutation carriers has the excess CGG repeats which bind and sequester proteins that are important for the appropriate function of the neurones. It is the sequestration of proteins or mRNA which probably leads to the RNA gain of function toxicity subsequently causal to FXTAS. These observations have been used to propose the 'toxic RNA gain of function model' to explain several disease states including myotonic dystrophy, Huntington-like disease type 2, and even possibly some forms of spinocerebellar ataxias (Cummings & Zoghbi 2000, Vincent et al. 2000).

Symptoms typically begin after age 50 in mostly male carriers, although an occasional female carrier may be affected (Hagerman et al. 2004). In a study of carriers in California, 17% of male carriers in their 50s had tremor and ataxia, 38% in their 60s, 47% in their 70s and 75% in their 80s (Jacquemont et al. 2004). Although some carriers may exhibit mild tremor or ataxia for decades, rare patients may rapidly progress to dementia. This variability in progression is probably related to secondary gene effects resulting in elevated mRNA or an additional independent mechanism for brain damage.

The existence of FXTAS brings new meaning to the issues of comorbidity because the same gene may be causing disease by a different molecular mechanism. On rare occasions, elements of both FXS and FXTAS may occur in the same individual. For instance, a person with the premutation can have mildly lowered levels of FMRP because of the mild translation deficit present in the premutation. This leads to anxiety or mild intellectual disability. The same individual may develop FXTAS later in life because of elevated mRNA and the inclusion neuropathology.

Conclusion

Given the new possibilities for attributing symptoms directly to specific genetic aberrations, many comorbid conditions once attributed to low intellectual functioning may actually be part of a specific behavioural cognitive phenotype unique to FXS or may be better understood as *molecular comorbidities* of FXS. The penetrance of specific behavioural cognitive symptoms probably depends on the interaction of FMRP with other genes through epistatic mechanisms. Some of these interactions may depend on sequence variations in epistatic genes.

In the last decade, researchers have successfully identified several genes that play modulatory roles in psychiatric disorders such as anxiety, mood instability and psychosis. Sequence variations in the serotonin transporter gene may determine if psychological stress results in affective disorder (Caspi et al. 2003), possibly via increased activation of the amygdala to fear-producing stimuli (Hariri et al. 2002). Schizophrenia, bipolar and obsessive-compulsive disorder may be modified by allelic variations in brain-derived neurotrophic factor (BDNF) (Neves-Pereira et al. 2002, Hall et al. 2003, Maier et al. 2003). Specific allelic gene variations in catechol O-methyltransferase (COMT), important in the metabolism of monoamines including dopamine, may determine psychosis and/or anxiety given the presence of other genetic vulnerability and environmental stressors (Enoch et al. 2003, Goldberg et al. 2003). However, these genes are not definitive in the determination of these psychiatric disorders but perhaps, when present in combination with a genetic defect like that found in FXS, lead to excessive anxiety.

To determine whether these genes interact with FMRP, one can isolate mRNA that binds specifically to FMRP. The binding of FMRP to unique mRNA probably regulates the translation of RNA to protein. There is preliminary evidence to suggest that FMRP may regulate BDNF (Castren et al. 2002), which has a known modulatory role in schizophrenia, bipolar and obsessive-compulsive disorder (Neves-Pereira et al. 2002, Hall et al. 2003, Fanous et al. 2004). Therefore a specific BDNF allele when present in individuals with FXS may result in affective instability with or without psychotic symptoms.

The concept of specific behavioural phenotypes characterising genetic syndromes has received much attention lately, even though, early on, specific behaviours were recognised as pathognomonic for certain syndromes: midline hand wringing in Rett syndrome or compulsive hyperphagia in Prader–Willi syndrome (PWS) (Denckla 2000, Moldavsky et al. 2001). Rett syndrome is uniquely included in the DSM-IV as a pervasive development disorder (PDD) (Moldavsky et al. 2001) even though current evidence suggests that the Rett behavioural phenotype is broader (Mount et al. 2003). Compulsive hyperphagia is one of the behaviours consistent with obsessive-compulsive disorder (OCD) that characterises PWS (Dimitropoulos et al. 2000). PWS set the precedent to consider a specific cognitive-behavioural phenotype in genetic disorders. Therefore, FXS phenotype should include psychiatric disorders. In fact, molecular overlap can lead to a Prader–Willi-like behavioural phenotype in fragile X. This subgroup of patients with FXS has severe hyperphagia, hypo-gonadism and obesity but a normal 15q region (Hagerman 2002). The CYFIP gene, which occurs at 15q in the Prader–Willi region, produces a protein that impacts closely with FMRP in the regulation of translation. It has been demonstrated that low expression of CYFIP is associated with the Prader–Willi-like phenotype in FXS (Nowicki et al. 2007).

More importantly, since the new molecular developments in FXS redefine how genetic abnormalities result in disease, other models of genetic manifestations of psychiatric disorder need to be considered. As mentioned earlier, the carrier state in females with the full mutation or males with the premutation was considered a 'normal' presentation without associated pathology (Hagerman & Hagerman 2004). New research has identified mild cognitive and/or behavioural deficits and schizoaffective traits in women who are carriers of the full mutation in addition to premature ovarian failure in women who have the pre-mutation. These are excellent examples of a young, healthy individual having onset of a disorder not related to ageing that may also be part of the FXS phenotype.

Given the various sub-phenotypes and molecular alterations that may be associated with FXS, the obvious question is how alterations in synapse formation that result in pervasive deficits in LTD and PPI can lead to such diverse behavioural manifestations, from intel-lectual disability, to autism, to schizophrenia, to premature ovarian failure, and lastly FXTAS. The answer may lie in understanding the impact of FMRP and mRNA alterations within a developmental framework.

Absence of FMRP early in development results in global intellectual impairment. Serotonin, which has been implicated in autism but without a clear aetiology, may alter the trajectory of FXS and manifest as anxiety as the individual matures, as described by Hessl and colleagues (2004b). Perhaps having a specific polymorphism of the serotonin transporter gene further aggravates the anxious state and results in autism (Muhle et al. 2004). Serotonin is thought to play a major role in shaping synaptic architecture throughout development (El-Mallakh et al. 2000). Furthermore, the serotonergic system interacts with BDNF, S100β and other chemical messengers including the GABAergic, glutamatergic and dopaminergic neurotransmitter systems (Sodhi & Sanders-Bush 2004).

Therefore, it would be plausible to suggest that a combination of primary defects in glutamatergic activity related to FMR1 gene dysfunction, coupled with mild alterations in serotonin activity and BDNF resulting in significant changes in LTD and PPI, may manifest as symptoms of autism in early childhood and psychosis later in early adolescence to mid-adult life. There is no question that the mechanisms proposed here to identify behavioural symptoms as part of the broader FXS phenotype rather than comorbidities of low intellectual function are speculative until more research occurs. However, the molecular methods to demonstrate their plausibility exist today. Rapid genotyping of individuals coupled with known behavioural associations of sequence variations of specific genes can be used to predict who may be more vulnerable to certain psychiatric comorbidities ranging from anxiety to autism to psychosis. Prediction of these risks will lead to more powerful prevention, intervention and treatment programmes to minimise the molecular comorbidities associated with the FXS such as autism, anxiety and specific cognitive dysfunction.

REFERENCES

Akshoomoff N, Pierce K, Courchesne E (2002) The neurobiological basis of autism from a developmental perspective. *Dev Psychopathol* **14**(3), 613–634.

Allingham-Hawkins DJ, Babul-Hirji R, Chitayat D et al. (1999) Fragile X premutation is a significant risk factor for premature ovarian failure: the International Collaborative POF in Fragile X Study – preliminary data. *Am J Med Genet* **83**, 322–325.

Amaral DG, Bauman MD, Schumann CM (2003) The amygdala and autism: implications from non–human primate studies. *Genes Brain Behav* **2**(5), 295–302.

Antar LN, Afroz R, Dictenberg JB, et al. (2004) Metabotropic glutamate receptor activation regulates fragile X mental retardation protein and FMR1 mRNA localization differentially in dendrites and at synapses. *J Neurosci* **24**(11), 2648–2655.

Ashworth A, Abusaad I, Walsh C, et al. (1996) Linkage analysis of the fragile X gene FMR-1 and schizophrenia: no evidence for linkage but report of a family with schizophrenia and an unstable triplet repeat. *Psychiatr Genet* **6**(2), 81–86.

Aziz M, Stathopulu E, Callias M, et al. (2003) Clinical features of boys with fragile X premutations and intermediate alleles. *Am J Med Genet* **121B**(1), 119–127.

Bailey DB Jr, Mesibov GB, Hatton DD et al. (1998) Autistic behavior in young boys with fragile X syndrome. *J Autism Dev Disord* **28**(6), 499–508.

Bailey DB Jr, Hatton DD, Skinner M, Mesibov GB (2001) Autistic behavior, FMR1 protein, and developmental trajectories in young males with fragile X syndrome. *J Autism Dev Disord* **31**(2), 165–174.

Bear MF, Huber KM, Warren ST (2004) The mGluR theory of fragile X mental retardation. *Trends Neurosci* **27**(7), 370–377.

Bell MV, Hirst M, Nakahori Y, et al. (1991) Physical mapping across the fragile X: hypermethylation and clinical expression of the fragile X syndrome. *Cell* **64**(4), 861–866.

Benassi G, Guarino M, Cammarat S, et al. (1990) An epidemiological study on severe mental retardation among schoolchildren in Bologna, Italy. *Dev Med Child Neurol* **32**(10), 895–901.

Berry-Kravis E, Potanos K (2004) Psychopharmacology in fragile X syndrome – present and future. *Ment Retard Dev Disabil Res Rev* **10**(1), 42–48.

Brainard SS, Schreiner RA, Hagerman RJ (1991) Cognitive profiles of the carrier fragile X woman. *Am J Med Genet* **38**(2–3), 505–508.

Brown V, Jin P, Ceman S, et al. (2001) Microarray identification of FMRP-associated brain mRNAs and altered mRNA translational profiles in fragile X syndrome. *Cell* **107**(4), 477–487.

Brown WT (2002) The molecular biology of the fragile X mutation. In: Hagerman RJ, Cronister A (eds) *The Fragile X Syndrome: Diagnosis, Treatment, and Research*. Baltimore: Johns Hopkins University Press.

Brown WT, Friedman E, Jenkins E, et al. (1982) Association of fragile X syndrome with autism. *Lancet* **1**(8263), 100.

Brunberg JA, Jaquemont S, Hagerman RJ, et al. (2002) Fragile X premutation carriers: characteristic MR imaging findings in adult males with progressive cerebellar and cognitive dysfunction. *Am J Neuroradiol* **23**(10), 1757–1766.

Carpenter NJ (1994) Genetic anticipation. Expanding tandem repeats. *Neurol Clin* **12**(4), 683–697.

Caspi A, Sugden K, Moffitt T, et al. (2003) Influence of life stress on depression: moderation by a polymorphism in the 5-HTT gene. *Science* **301**(5631), 386–389.

Castren M, Lampinen K, Miettinen R, et al. (2002) BDNF regulates the expression of fragile X mental retardation protein mRNA in the hippocampus. *Neurobiol Dis* **11**(1), 221–229.

Chen LS, Tassone F, Sahota P, Hagerman P (2003) The (CGG)n repeat element within the 5′ untranslated region of the FMR1 message provides both positive and negative cis effects on in vivo translation of a downstream reporter. *Hum Mol Genet* **12**(23), 3067–3074.

Cornish KM, Turk J, Wilding J, et al. (2004) Annotation: deconstructing the attention deficit in fragile X syndrome: a developmental neuropsychological approach. *J Child Psychol Psychiatr* **45**(6), 1042–1053.

Cummings CJ, Zoghbi HY (2000) Trinucleotide repeats: mechanisms and pathophysiology. *Annu Rev Genom Hum Genet* **1**, 281–328.

Denckla MB (2000) Overview: specific behavioral/cognitive phenotypes of genetic disorders. *Ment Retard Dev Disabil Res Rev* **6**(2), 81–83.

Dimitropoulos A, Feurer I, Roof E, et al. (2000) Appetitive behavior, compulsivity, and neurochemistry in Prader–Willi syndrome. *Ment Retard Dev Disabil Res Rev* **6**(2), 125–130.

Einfeld SL, Tonge BJ (1996) Population prevalence of psychopathology in children and adolescents with intellectual disability: II. Epidemiological findings. *J Intellect Disabil Res* **40**(Pt 2), 99–109.

Eliez S, Blasey C, Freund L, et al. (2001) Brain anatomy, gender and IQ in children and adolescents with fragile X syndrome. *Brain* **124**(Pt 8), 1610–1618.

El-Mallakh RS, Peters C, Waltrip C (2000) Antidepressant treatment and neural plasticity. *J Child Adolesc Psychopharmacol* **10**(4), 287–294.

Enoch MA, Xu K, Ferro E, et al. (2003) Genetic origins of anxiety in women: a role for a functional catechol-O-methyltransferase polymorphism. *Psychiatr Genet* **13**(1), 33–41.

Fanous AH, Neale M, Straub R, et al. (2004) Clinical features of psychotic disorders and polymorphisms in HT2A, DRD2, DRD4, SLC6A3 (DAT1), and BDNF: a family based association study. *Am J Med Genet* **125B**(1), 69–78.

Feinstein C, Reiss AL (1998) Autism: the point of view from fragile X studies. *J Autism Dev Disord* **28**(5), 393–405.

Frankland PW, Wang Y, Rosner B, et al. (2004) Sensorimotor gating abnormalities in young males with fragile X syndrome and Fmr1-knockout mice. *Mol Psychiatr* **9**(4), 417–425.

Freund LS, Reiss AL, Abrams MT (1993) Psychiatric disorders associated with fragile X in the young female. *Pediatrics* **91**(2), 321–329.

Fu YH, Kuhl D, Pizzuti A, et al. (1991) Variation of the CGG repeat at the fragile X site results in genetic instability: resolution of the Sherman paradox. *Cell* **67**(6), 1047–1058.

Garrett AS, Menon V, MacKenzie K, Reiss AL (2004) Here's looking at you, kid: neural systems underlying face and gaze processing in fragile X syndrome. *Arch Gen Psychiatr* **61**(3), 281–288.

Goldberg TE, Egan F, Gscheidle T, et al. (2003) Executive subprocesses in working memory: relationship to catechol-O-methyltransferase Val158Met genotype and schizophrenia. *Arch Gen Psychiatr* **60**(9), 889–896.

Goodlin-Jones BL, Tassone F, Gane LW, Hagerman RJ (2004) Autistic spectrum disorder and the fragile X premutation. *J Dev Behav Pediatr* **25**(6), 392–398.

Greco C, Hagerman R, Tassone F, et al. (2002) Neuronal intranuclear inclusions in a new cerebellar tremor/ataxia syndrome among fragile X carriers. *Brain* **125**(8), 1760–1771.

Guerreiro MM, Camargo E, Kato M, et al. (1998) Fragile X syndrome. Clinical, electroencephalographic and neuroimaging characteristics. *Arq Neuropsiquiatr* **56**(1), 18–23.

Hagerman RJ (2002) Physical and behavioral phenotype. In: Hagerman RJ, Cronister A (eds) *The Fragile X Syndrome: Diagnosis, Treatment, and Research*. Baltimore: Johns Hopkins University Press.

Hagerman PJ, Hagerman RJ (2002) *Fragile X Syndrome: Diagnosis, Treatment, and Research*, 3rd edn. Baltimore: Johns Hopkins University Press.

Hagerman PJ, Hagerman RJ (2004) The fragile-X premutation: a maturing perspective. *Am J Hum Genet* **74**(5), 805–816.

Hagerman RJ, Staley L, O'Conner R, et al. (1996) Learning-disabled males with a fragile X CGG expansion in the upper premutation size range. *Pediatrics* **97**(1), 122–126.

Hagerman RJ, Leehey M, Heinrichs W, et al. (2001) Intention tremor, parkinsonism, and generalized brain atrophy in male carriers of fragile X. *Neurology* **57**, 127–130.

Hagerman RJ, Leavitt B, Farzin F, et al. (2004) Fragile X associated tremor/ataxia syndrome (FXTAS) in females with the FMR1 premutation. *Am J Hum Genet* **74**(5), 1051–1056.

Hall D, Dhilla A, Charalambous A, et al. (2003) Sequence variants of the brain-derived neurotrophic factor (BDNF) gene are strongly associated with obsessive-compulsive disorder. *Am J Hum Genet* **73**(2), 370–376.

Hardan A, Sahl R. (1997) Psychopathology in children and adolescents with developmental disorders. *Res Dev Disabil* **18**(5), 369–382.

Hariri AR, Mattay VS, Tessitore A, et al. (2002) Serotonin transporter genetic variation and the response of the human amygdala. *Science* **297**(5580), 400–403.

Harrison PJ, Weinberger DR (2004) Schizophrenia genes, gene expression, and neuropathology: on the matter of their convergence. *Mol Psychiatr* **10**(1), 40–68.

Hessl D, Dyer-Friedman J, Glaser B, et al. (2001) The influence of environmental and genetic factors on behavior problems and autistic symptoms in boys and girls with fragile X syndrome. *Pediatrics* **108**(5), e88.

Hessl D, Glaser B, Dyer-Friedman J, et al. (2002) Cortisol and behavior in fragile X syndrome. *Psychoneuroendocrinology* **27**, 855–872.

Hessl D, Rivera SM, Reiss AL (2004a) The neuroanatomy and neuroendocrinology of fragile X syndrome. *Ment Retard Dev Disabil Res Rev* **10**(1), 17–24.

Hessl D, Cohen S, Perry H, Tassone F, Hagerman RJ (2004b) Potentiated startle and galvanic skin responses to social and emotional stimuli in children with fragile X: a pilot study. Paper presented at the International Fragile X Conference, Washington, DC.

Jacquemont S, Hagerman RJ, Leehey M, et al. (2003) Fragile X premutation tremor/ataxia syndrome: molecular, clinical, and neuroimaging correlates. *Am J Hum Genet* **72**, 869–878.

Jacquemont S, Hagerman RJ, Leehey MA, et al. (2004) Penetrance of the fragile X-associated tremor/ataxia syndrome (FXTAS) in a premutation carrier population: initial results from a California family-based study. *JAMA* **291**(4), 460–469.

Jamain S, Betancur C, Quach H, et al. (2002) Linkage and association of the glutamate receptor 6 gene with autism. *Mol Psychiatr* **7**(3), 302–310.

Jansen LM, Gispen-de Weid CC, van der Gaag RJ, et al. (2003) Differentiation between autism and multiple complex developmental disorder in response to psychosocial stress. *Neuropsychopharmacology* **28**(3), 582–590.

Jin P, Zarnescu DC, Zhang F, et al. (2003) RNA-mediated neurodegeneration caused by the Fragile X premutation r CGG repeats in *Drosophila*. *Neuron* **39**, 739–747.

Kemper MB, Hagerman RJ, Ahmad RS, et al. (1986) Cognitive profiles and the spectrum of clinical manifestations in heterozygous fra (X) females. *Am J Med Genet* **23**(1–2), 139–156.

Kremer EJ, Pritchard M, Lynch M, et al. (1991) Mapping of DNA instability at the fragile X to a trinucleotide repeat sequence p(CCG)n. *Science* **252**(5013), 1711–1714.

Kumra S, Giedd JN, Vaituzis AC, et al. (2000) Childhood-onset psychotic disorders: magnetic resonance imaging of volumetric differences in brain structure. *Am J Psychiatr* **157**(9), 1467–1474.

Lachiewicz AM (1992) Abnormal behaviors of young girls with fragile X syndrome. *Am J Med Genet* **43**(1–2), 72–77.

Lachiewicz AM, Dawson DV (1994) Behavior problems of young girls with fragile X syndrome: factor scores on the Conners' Parent's Questionnaire. *Am J Med Genet* **51**(4), 364–369.

Le Pen G, Moreau JL (2002) Disruption of prepulse inhibition of startle reflex in a neurodevelopmental model of schizophrenia: reversal by clozapine, olanzapine and risperidone but not by haloperidol. *Neuropsychopharmacology* **27**(1), 1–11.

Loesch DZ, Huggins RM, Hagerman RJ (2004) Phenotypic variation and FMRP levels in fragile X. *Ment Retard Dev Disabil Res Rev* **10**(1), 31–41.

Lubs HA (1969) A marker X chromosome. *Am J Human Genet* **21**, 231–244.

Maier W, Zobel A, Rietschel M (2003) Genetics of schizophrenia and affective disorders. *Pharmacopsychiatry* **36**(Suppl 3), S195–202.

Margolis RL, Abraham MR, Gatchell SB, et al. (1997) cDNAs with long CAG trinucleotide repeats from human brain. *Hum Genet* **100**(1), 114–122.

McAlonan GM, Daly E, Kumari V, et al. (2002) Brain anatomy and sensorimotor gating in Asperger's syndrome. *Brain* **125**(Pt 7), 1594–1606.

McCarley RW, Wible CG, Frumin M, et al. (1999) MRI anatomy of schizophrenia. *Biol Psychiatr* **45**(9), 1099–1119.

McCracken JT, McGough J, Shah B, et al. (2002) Risperidone in children with autism and serious behavioral problems. *N Engl J Med* **347**(5), 314–321.

Miller LJ, McIntosh DN, McGrath J, et al. (1999) Electrodermal responses to sensory stimuli in individuals with fragile X syndrome: a preliminary report. *Am J Med Genet* **83**, 268–279.

Moldavsky M, Lev D, Lerman-Sagie T (2001) Behavioral phenotypes of genetic syndromes: a reference guide for psychiatrists. *J Am Acad Child Adolesc Psychiatr* **40**(7), 749–761.

Mount RH, Hastings RP, Reilly S, et al. (2003) Towards a behavioral phenotype for Rett syndrome. *Am J Ment Retard* **108**(1), 1–12.

Muhle R, Trentacoste SV, Rapin I (2004) The genetics of autism. *Pediatrics* **113**(5), e472–486.

Munir F, Cornish KM, Wilding J (2000) A neuropsychological profile of attention deficits in young males with fragile X syndrome. *Neuropsychologia* **38**(9), 1261–1270.

Neves-Pereira M, Mundo E, Muglia P, et al. (2002) The brain-derived neurotrophic factor gene confers susceptibility to bipolar disorder: evidence from a family-based association study. *Am J Hum Genet* **71**(3), 651–655.

Nolin SL, Glicksman A, Houck GE, et al. (1994) Mosaicism in fragile X affected males. *Am J Med Genet* **51**(4), 509–512.

Nowicki ST, Tassone F, Ono MY et al. (2007) The Prader-Willi Phenotype of Fragile X Syndrome. *J Dev Behav Pediatr* 28, 133–138.

O'Donovan MC, Guy C, Craddok N, et al. (1995) Expanded CAG repeats in schizophrenia and bipolar disorder. *Nat Genet* **10**(4), 380–381.

O'Donnell WT, Warren ST (2002) A decade of molecular studies of fragile S syndrome. *Annu Rev Neurosci* **25**, 315–338.

Otani S, Daniel H, Roisin MP, et al. (2003) Dopaminergic modulation of long-term synaptic plasticity in rat prefrontal neurons. *Cereb Cortex* **13**(11), 1251–1256.

Petronis A, Kennedy JL (1995) Unstable genes – unstable mind? *Am J Psychiatr* **152**(2), 164–172.

Philofsky A, Hepburn SL, Hayes A, et al. (2004) Linguistic and cognitive functioning and autism symptoms in young children with fragile X syndrome. *Am J Ment Retard* **109**(3), 208–218.

Pierce K, Haist F, Sedaghat F, Courchesne E (2004) The brain response to personally familiar faces in autism: findings of fusiform activity and beyond. *Brain* **127**(Pt 12), 2703–2716.

Pietrobono R, Tabolacci E, Zaifa F, et al. (2005) Molecular dissection of the events leading to inactivation of the FMR1 gene. *Hum Mol Genet* **14**(2), 267–277.

Prosser H, Moss, S, Costello H, et al. (1998) Reliability and validity of the Mini PAS-ADD for assessing psychiatric disorders in adults with intellectual disability. *J Intellect Disabil Res* **42**(Pt 4), 264–272.

Purcell AE, Jeon OH, Zimmerman AW, et al. (2001) Postmortem brain abnormalities of the glutamate neurotransmitter system in autism. *Neurology* **57**(9), 1618–1628.

Reiss AL, Lee J, Freund L (1994) Neuroanatomy of fragile X syndrome: the temporal lobe. *Neurology* **44**(7), 1317–1324.

Richdale AL, Prior MR (1992) Urinary cortisol circadian rhythm in a group of high-functioning children with autism. *J Autism Dev Disord* **22**(3), 433–447.

Riddle JE, Cheema A, Sobesky WE, et al. (1998) Phenotypic involvement in females with the FMR1 gene mutation. *Am J Ment Retard* **102**(6), 590–601.

Rivera SM, Menon V, White CD, et al. (2002) Functional brain activation during arithmetic processing in females with fragile X syndrome is related to FMR1 protein expression. *Hum Brain Mapp* **16**(4), 206–218.

Roberts JE, Boccia ML, Bailey DB Jr., et al. (2001) Cardiovascular indices of physiological arousal in boys with fragile X syndrome. *Dev Psychobiol* **39**(2), 107–123.

Rogers SJ, Wehner DE, Hagerman R (2001) The behavioral phenotype in fragile X: symptoms of autism in very young children with fragile X syndrome, idiopathic autism, and other developmental disorders. *J Dev Behav Pediatr* **22**(6), 409–417.

Ross CA, McInnis MG, Margolis RL, et al. (1993) Genes with triplet repeats: candidate mediators of neuropsychiatric disorders. *Trends Neurosci* **16**(7), 254–260.

Rousseau F (1994) The fragile X syndrome: implications of molecular genetics for the clinical syndrome. *Eur J Clin Invest* **24**(1), 1–10.

Schumann CM, Hamstra J, Goodlin-Jones BL, et al. (2004) The amygdala is enlarged in children but not adolescents with autism: the hippocampus is enlarged at all ages. *J Neurosci* **24**(28), 6392–6401.

Serajee FJ, et al. (2003) The metabotropic glutamate receptor 8 gene at 7q31: partial duplication and possible association with autism. *J Med Genet* **40**(4), e42.

Simon TJ, et al. (2005) Visuospatial and numerical cognitive deficits in children with Chromosome 22q11.2 Deletion Syndrome. *Cortex* **41**, 131–141.

Siomi H, Ishizuka A, Siomi MC (2004) RNA interference: a new mechanism by which FMRP acts in the normal brain? What can Drosophila teach us? *Ment Retard Dev Disabil Res Rev* **10**(1), 68–74.

Sobesky WE, et al. (1996) Molecular-clinical correlations in females with fragile X. *Am J Med Genet* **64**(2), 340–345.

Sodhi MS, Sanders-Bush E (2004) Serotonin and brain development. *Int Rev Neurobiol* **59**, 111–174.

Tassone F, Hagerman RJ, Iklé DN, et al. (1999) FMRP expression as a potential prognostic indicator in fragile X syndrome. *Am J Med Genet* **84**(3), 250–261.

Tassone F, Hagerman RJ, Taylor AK, et al. (2000a) Clinical involvement and protein expression in individuals with the FMR1 premutation. *Am J Med Genet* **91**, 144–152.

Tassone F, Hagerman RJ, Taylor AK, et al. (2000b) Elevated levels of FMR1 mRNA in carrier males: a new mechanism of involvement in the fragile-X syndrome. *Am J Hum Genet* **66**(1), 6–15.

Todd PK, Mack KJ, Malter JS (2003) The fragile X mental retardation protein is required for type-I metabotropic glutamate receptor-dependent translation of PSD-95. *Proc Natl Acad Sci USA* **100**(24), 14374–14378.

Tsuang MT, Stone WS, Faraone SV (2000) Toward reformulating the diagnosis of schizophrenia. *Am J Psychiatr* **157**(7), 1041–1050.

Turner G, Eastman C, Casey J, et al. (1975) X-linked mental retardation associated with macro-orchidism. *J Med Genet* **12**(4), 367–371.

Verkerk AJ, Pieretti M, Sutcliffe JS, et al. (1991) Identification of a gene (FMR-1) containing a CGG repeat coincident with a breakpoint cluster region exhibiting length variation in fragile X syndrome. *Cell* **65**(5), 905–914.

Vincent A, Heitz D, Petit C, et al. (1991) Abnormal pattern detected in fragile-X patients by pulsed-field gel electrophoresis. *Nature* **349**(6310), 624–626.

Vincent JB, Paterson AD, Strong E, et al. (2000) The unstable trinucleotide repeat story of major psychosis. *Am J Med Genet* **97**(1), 77–97.

Wilding J, Cornish K, Munir F (2002) Further delineation of the executive deficit in males with fragile-X syndrome. *Neuropsychologia* **40**(8), 1343–1349.

8
CHANNELOPATHIES

Sameer M Zuberi

Ion channels are specialised transmembrane proteins that are essential for controlling electrical signalling and neurotransmitter release throughout the nervous system. When comorbid neurological or behavioural disorders affect an individual, the explanation may be found in a single ion channel mutation producing pathology in different tissues. The epilepsies are the most common serious neurological disorders and the last decade has taught us that they are largely a family of ion channelopathies. The comorbidities that exist alongside epilepsy such as learning and behaviour problems, migraine and movement disorders may also have their basis in the dysfunction of the channel producing the epilepsy. The genetic mutation provides a way in which the clinician and molecular biologist can research and understand these relationships. The study of channelopathies is proving new insights into the epileptic encephalopathies, an important and potentially treatable cause of learning and behaviour problems in childhood.

In the last two decades more than 40 neurological channelopathies have been described (Zuberi 2003). The majority of these disorders have a genetic basis and are single-gene syndromes within common classes of neurological disorders such as epilepsy, movement disorders and migraine. The study of monogenic channelopathies has resulted in important insights into these common disorders with complex inheritance which are the bread and butter of the neurologist's practice. In this chapter I use two groups of channelopathies, the primary episodic ataxias and the SCN1A (sodium ion channel)-related epileptic encephalopathies, to illustrate how clinical and basic science research can explain many of the comorbidities seen in neurological practice.

It is over 50 years since Hodgkin and Huxley first described the generation of the nerve action potential in the squid giant axon (Hodgkin & Huxley 1952). They determined that the electrical impulses were generated by the rapid passage of ions across the cell membrane through what they termed 'active patches'. We now call these patches ion channels and know that they are large macromolecular proteins which span the cell membrane.

Hodgkin and Huxley were able to mathematically deduce three of the key properties of ion channels: that they have a central aqueous pore through which the ions pass, that the pore can be rapidly opened and closed (gated) and that the channels are specific to different ion species. The development of patch clamp techniques to measure current across single channels in the 1970s, the advances in molecular biology of the 1980s which allowed the amino acid sequence of channel proteins to be described, and the beautiful 3-D pictures of bacterial potassium channels from X-ray crystallography in the 1990s have all confirmed these properties (Neher & Sakman 1976, Hille et al. 1999).

There are two major classes of ion channels: voltage gated and ligand gated. Ion channels can be regarded as excitable molecules which allow passage of ions through changes in conformation in response to a variety of stimuli. The action potential along a nerve is transmitted by the sequential depolarisation and repolarisation of the cell membrane by the passage of sodium and potassium ions across the membrane. Changes in membrane voltage cause voltage-gated sodium channels to open, allowing a rapid influx of ions across the membrane with resultant depolarisation. This change in membrane voltage leads to the opening of potassium channels and the rapid passage of potassium ions out of the cell, resulting in repolarisation of the membrane. When the action potential reaches the neuromuscular junction, a sequence of events leads to release of acetylcholine (the ligand) which binds to the acetylcholine receptor, a ligand-gated ion channel, on the postsynaptic membrane. The binding of the ligand leads to a change in conformation of the protein and opening of the channel, allowing sodium ions to pass across the membrane and set in motion the train of events leading to muscle contraction.

Many of the channelopathies are paroxysmal disorders. The ion channel mutation may impair channel function to a degree that only becomes significant when there are additional factors which affect channel function. These factors include temperature, the pH surrounding the channel, intracellular messengers and many other aspects of the channel environment (Hille 2001). In some disorders chronic channel dysfunction can result in progressive impairment of function and interictal signs and symptoms.

The emergence of the channelopathies has benefited from the recent rapid advances in molecular biology. Mutations identified in humans can be incorporated into ion channel gene cDNA, the mutant channel expressed in a cell membrane and the current across the mutant channel measured. These functional studies not only provide insight into the basic physiology of disease but may suggest novel therapeutic pathways. The channelopathies are therefore an important source for translational research.

The primary episodic ataxias
Episodic ataxias type 1 and 2 are both rare autosomal dominant channelopathies in which there is good clinical and physiological evidence that the primary pathological disturbance is of cerebellar function. However, ion channel dysfunction in other tissues may present as a variety of other problems.

EPISODIC ATAXIA TYPE 1
Episodic ataxia type 1 (EA1) is caused by mutations in the *KCNA1* gene which codes for the Kv1.1 potassium ion channel (Browne et al. 1994). The widespread expression of this channel in cerebellum, cerebral cortex and peripheral nerve helps explain the symptoms associated with this disorder. EA1 usually has its onset in childhood and is characterised by episodes of cerebellar ataxia and dysarthria lasting seconds to minutes triggered by startle, sudden movement or emotion. The other key clinical feature is interictal myokymia, also termed neuromyotonia. Some individuals describe a brief aura before the event,

such as a rising sensation up the body, warning them that they will have to hold onto something for support. The ataxia may be associated with a coarse tremor and the movements may have features of chorea or dystonia. In between attacks there is no interictal ataxia.

Myokymia, the clinical sign most useful in making the diagnosis, may be subtle and missed if not looked for specifically. The failure of normal cell membrane repolarisation through the dysfunctional potassium channels results in peripheral nerve hyperexcitability and continuous motor unit action potentials. This is seen clinically as myokymia which is best observed as semi-rhythmic side-to-side movements of the fingers with the hands outstretched or as rippling of the muscles of the lower eyelid. Continuous motor unit activity can be demonstrated by surface electromyography without the necessity for needle insertion.

Peripheral nerve hyperexcitability can be prominent in early infancy with neuromyotonia resulting in fisting of hands, non-fixed contractures and later toe walking. One family I have studied included two members diagnosed after birth as having an atypical arthrogryposis (Zuberi et al. 1999). In rare families generalised myokymia may be present without any history of episodic ataxia. We have termed this familial generalised myokymia (Eunson et al. 2000). The proband of a Scottish family had no symptoms apart from intermittent toe walking until he presented with generalised neuromyotonia in a vomiting illness aged 3. Spontaneous rippling movements and hypertrophy of larger muscles in the limbs were more obvious in this child from mid childhood onwards. This was the first report of isolated neuromyotonia caused by a genetic defect in this potassium channel.

In 1997 we first reported a family with EA1 in which two individuals had epilepsy as well as the movement disorder (Zuberi et al. 1999). Reviewing the literature, we discovered that about 10% of published cases with EA1 have epileptic seizures. The epileptic seizures in EA1 are focal seizures with impairment of consciousness, sometimes with secondary generalisation. The proband in this family presented with epileptic apnoeas akin to events in benign neonatal and infantile epileptic syndromes. This rare movement disorder was providing early insights into the pathogenesis of infantile epilepsies. In 1998 autosomal dominant benign familial neonatal convulsions were first associated with mutations in two other potassium channel subunits: KCNQ2 and KCNQ3 (Biervert et al. 1998, Charlier et al. 1998).

Dysfunction of a potassium channel in the cerebral cortex can cause epilepsy, dysfunction in the cerebellum can cause episodic ataxia and dysfunction in peripheral nerve can cause myokymia and muscle hypertrophy. Why should some families have more than one tissue significantly involved whereas others have milder symptoms? Clues can be found in the functional study of the specific mutations (Eunson et al. 2000). Both mutant channels could be successfully expressed in *Xenopus* oocyte. The current amplitude was significantly reduced through the mutant channel from the EA1 and epilepsy family (Zuberi 1999). The current amplitude was normal in the generalised myokymia family but other studies on the time course of deactivation on membrane repolarisation showed abnormalities compared to the wild type (Eunson et al. 2000). These changes were relatively subtle compared to those in the EA1 and epilepsy mutant channels. Therefore, a more severe functional impairment appears to be associated with more widespread tissue involvement and a more severe phenotype.

Further evidence that Kv1.1 potassium channels are important in the pathogenesis of epilepsy and neuromyotonia comes from autoimmune limbic encephalitis. In this condition there is evidence of autoantibodies against the Kv1.1 channels (Vincent et al. 2004). These channels are expressed in the limbic system and autoimmune attack can result in epileptic seizures, encephalopathy and long-term cognitive impairment. Another feature seen in some individuals with limbic encephalitis is myokymia, indicating antibody-mediated attack on channels in peripheral nerve. Awareness of this disorder is important as it can be misdiagnosed as herpes simplex encephalitis and it may respond to immunotherapy.

Another disorder in which potassium channel dysfunction can explain apparently unrelated comorbidities is the Jervell and Lange-Nielsen syndrome (LQTS1). This condition may present to the neurologist in the first seizure/epilepsy clinic as a cause of loss of consciousness. This is not an epilepsy syndrome but the association of a cardiac arrhythmia – long QT syndrome – and sensorineural deafness. Mutations in a potassium channel gene KCNQ1 cause both the arrhythmia and the deafness (Wang et al. 1996). The potassium channels are important in maintaining a specific potassium concentration in the endolymph of the cochlea. The mechanisms in which cardiac arrhythmias are produced are similar to epilepsy. The KCNQ1 channel is expressed in the heart and is closely linked to KCNQ2 and 3 which are expressed in the brain and associated with neonatal epilepsy.

EPISODIC ATAXIA TYPE 2

Episodic ataxia type 2 (EA2) is the most common of the paroxysmal ataxias and is associated with mutations in the *CACNA1A* gene which codes for the α subunit of a voltage-gated calcium channel (Ophoff et al. 1996). EA2 is allelic with familial hemiplegic migraine (a variant of migraine with aura) and spinocerebellar ataxia type 6 (a late-onset slowly progressive ataxia). These are three distinct conditions but phenotypic overlap may occur. In contrast to EA1, the episodes of ataxia in EA2 are much longer, lasting hours. Individuals with EA2 can have interictal cerebellar signs and a slowly progressive background ataxia. Onset of symptoms is typically in childhood. Triggers for the ataxic episodes include physical and emotional stress. This includes startle, movement and anxiety. Gait ataxia may be accompanied by dysarthria, nystagmus, vertigo, nausea and headache. Acetazolamide may be dramatically effective in EA2, so much so that it has been termed acetazolamide-responsive ataxia (Griggs et al. 1978). About 50% of EA2 patients report headaches which fulfil the diagnostic criteria for migraine. The headache can have features of a hemiplegic migraine.

Gaze-evoked nystagmus may be present between attacks but interictal cerebellar signs may be difficult to demonstrate. Failure to suppress the vestibulo-ocular reflex with fixation may be the only early sign of cerebellar vermis dysfunction. With time, spontaneous vertical nystagmus may become evident, magnetic resonance imaging (MRI) may reveal subtle vermian atrophy and MR spectroscopy can show an alkaline cerebellar pH (Jen et al. 2007). Channel dysfunction can therefore cause chronic and progressive symptoms as well as paroxysmal events.

In 2001 we reported a single case of a boy with EA2, intellectual disability and epileptic absences (Jouvenceau et al. 2001). A heterozygous novel stop mutation was identified in the CACNA1A gene. Functional studies showed that there was a markedly reduced current through the mutant channel and that the current was lower than seen with other EA2-causing mutations. The mutation in heterozygous models also seemed to reduce the expression of the normal channels in the cell membrane. The comparative severity of this mutation might explain why this boy had ataxia, absence epilepsy and intellectual disability. That calcium channels might be implicated in one of the most common idiopathic epilepsy subtypes, absence epilepsy, had been suggested by spontaneously occurring mouse mutants such as totterer who have mutations in the homologous murine calcium channel to human CACNA1A (Fletcher & Frankel 1999). These mice have epileptic absences and cerebellar ataxia. Following the first single case report, families with absence epilepsy and episodic ataxia have been reported. In one family with five affected individuals, it was notable that one child with absences developed marked cerebellar ataxia when he was on antiepileptic medications (Imbrici et al. 2004). This suggests that the mutation causing the epilepsy can also make an individual vulnerable to the side effects of medication and determine the nature of the side effect, in this case ataxia.

Dravet syndrome and other SCN1A-related infantile epileptic encephalopathies

Dravet syndrome, also known as severe myoclonic epilepsy in infancy (SMEI), is a severe form of infantile-onset epilepsy first described in 1978 (Dravet 1978). This is an epilepsy seen by all child neurologists with a distinct pattern of seizure types and temporal evolution but with variable EEG features (Dravet et al. 1992). In 2001 Claes et al. showed that the syndrome is associated with *de novo* mutations in the gene encoding for the α1 subunit of the neuronal sodium channel – SCN1A. The majority of infants with SCN1A-related epilepsies go on to experience most, if not all, of the serious morbidities associated with epilepsy, including refractory seizures, convulsive and non-convulsive status epilepticus, intellectual disability, speech and behaviour problems and progressive motor impairment.

Identification of the genetic basis of Dravet syndrome has allowed the detailed study of the variation in presentation of infantile epilepsies associated with mutations in SCN1A. This has led to further suggested subclassifications of Dravet syndrome/SMEI which I regard as variably helpful and at times confusing. Several phenotypes have been described as borderline or borderland Dravet or SMEI. These include intractable childhood epilepsy with generalised tonic clonic seizures (ICEGTCS), SMEB (borderland SMEB), SMEB-M (without myoclonus), SMEB-SW (without generalised spike and wave), and SMEB-O (SMEB lacking more than one typical SMEI characteristic) (Fujiwara et al. 2003, Harkin 2007).

My clinical impression and experience from reviewing the clinical details of more than 800 cases referred to the Glasgow SCN1A molecular genetic diagnostic service in the last 3 years is that the borderline Dravet/SMEI phenotypes overlap each other so much that in reality they are best classed as one group – borderline Dravet. In my view and that of several authors, classic Dravet syndrome or SMEI does not necessarily include myoclonus (Depienne et al. 2008, Dravet et al. 1992). For ease of reference I call the two groups together

Dravet Syndrome and if subdivided, Dravet-C (classic) and Dravet-B (Borderline). SCNIA mutations may be very rarely related to other severe epilepsy phenotypes including Lennox–Gastaut, severe infantile multifocal epilepsy and infantile spasms. More common SCN1A associations, though significantly less common than with Dravet, are with less severe phenotypes found in families with genetic (generalised) epilepsy with febrile seizures.

Dravet syndrome is well suited to translational research work. It presents in the first year of life, typically in children with no pre-existing developmental problems who go on to develop several different seizure types including status epilepticus. Seizure types within Dravet syndrome such as status epilepticus may be life threatening and sudden unexpected death in epilepsy can occur. There is a well-recognised and significant mortality associated with the syndrome which may extend into other SCN1A-related epilepsies (Dravet et al. 2002, Hindocha et al. 2008). SCN1A is expressed in cardiac muscle but it has not to date been shown to be associated with cardiac arrhythmias.

Inherent in the concept of an epileptic encephalopathy is the idea that controlling the epileptic seizures and abnormal electrical activity in the brain can improve development and behaviour. The knowledge that most cases of Dravet syndrome are associated with mutations in SCN1A has allowed the study of genotype/phenotype relationships in epilepsy in addition to research on seizure-generating mechanisms using functional studies and mouse models (Ragsdale 2008). The majority of SCN1A gene mutations cause a loss of function, though they can sometimes cause a gain of function. A loss of function can predispose to epileptic seizures as these channels are widely expressed on inhibitory GABA interneurones. Dysfunctional channels would cause a failure of inhibition in the nervous system.

Epileptic seizures in almost all children begin before 1 year of age. The onset is characterised by prolonged (>20 minutes) generalised clonic or hemi-clonic seizures often resulting in status epilepticus and intensive care unit (ICU) admission. In 60–70% of cases they are triggered by fever or elevated temperature such as immersion in a hot bath (Ohki et al. 1997). The first seizure may be around the time of the first immunisations in infancy and Dravet syndrome may be misdiagnosed as vaccine encephalopathy (Berkovic et al. 2006). Recurrent admissions to the ICU are not exceptional.

In the first year of life the EEG is usually normal, as is development. In some cases generalised spike and wave bursts or focal slow-wave activity may be seen. If photosensitivity is detected in a child with recurrent prolonged febrile seizures in infancy, this is suggestive of a diagnosis of Dravet syndrome. In the first 139 cases of SCN1A mutation-positive Dravet syndrome referred to the Glasgow Epilepsy Genetic Service, 19 (14%) were reported to have photosensitivity. In the second year of life a variety of seizure types can begin. These include afebrile generalised tonic-clonic, generalised clonic, myoclonic, focal and atypical absence seizures. The presence of different seizure types has led Dravet syndrome to be termed severe polymorphous or polymorphic epilepsy in infancy.

The distinctive feature of Dravet syndrome is the temporal evolution with typically refractory epileptic seizures of various types from the second year. The clinical expression of the ion channel function is dependent on the rest of the individual's genetic background, environmental factors and specific tissue expression of the mutant channels but also on the developmental stage of the child. It is some time in the second or third year that it becomes clear that the child is not developing normally. All aspects of learning are affected to a variable degree (Cassé-Perrot et al. 2001). The infant may acquire their first words at about a year of age but subsequent language development can be severely affected, with many children losing even these few words. Behaviour in early childhood is often characterised by poor attention and concentration with related hyperactivity. The literature suggests that the more frequent the seizures are in the first 2 years, the worse the subsequent learning and behaviour problems are. Some children develop autistic features. Dravet syndrome is therefore characterised by a true epileptic encephalopathy.

Motor development may be adversely affected with gait ataxia and subsequent development of pyramidal signs. It is likely that SCNIA is expressed on GABA inhibitory interneurones in the cerebellum as well as the cerebral cortex. As well as ataxia, limb dystonia and true spasticity may develop. As well as chronic ataxia and dystonia, paroxysmal movement disorders may also occur (Ohtsuka et al. 2003).

Despite trials of many antiepileptic medications, seizures usually continue, typically several per day. If the syndromic diagnosis is not considered, the severe epilepsy and neurological deterioration may result in the child having extensive investigations including neuroimaging, metabolic and invasive tests such as lumbar punctures and muscle biopsies. Early genetic diagnosis can prevent morbidity from unnecessary invasive investigations. The Glasgow Epilepsy Genetic Service uses a joint clinical and molecular genetic approach with a clinical referral form screened by a child neurologist prior to genetic testing. With this approach, we have an approximately 30% mutation detection rate. The peak age for genetic diagnosis in Glasgow is between 1 and 2 years, i.e. before the full syndrome has developed. This early diagnosis provides hope that earlier, more effective treatment may prevent or reduce some of the morbidity associated with the syndrome. It may also prevent misdiagnosis as vaccine encephalopathy.

The most exciting development in terms of therapy relates to the use of stiripentol. A randomised controlled trial and a meta-analysis of all medication trials in Dravet syndrome suggest that stiripentol can be highly effective in controlling epileptic seizures (Chiron et al. 2000, Kassai et al. 2008). The medication has at least two mode of actions which may be relevant *in vivo*. It inhibits the metabolism of benzodiazepines and valproate, thus raising drug levels, and it also has a positive effect on GABA transmission. The effectiveness of stiripentol and the knowledge of the genetic defect will suggest novel therapeutic possibilities for the syndrome.

Early anecdotal information and my clinical experience suggest that aggressive targeted therapy of Dravet syndrome after an early genetic diagnosis can lead to improved seizure control and reduction in the severity of the epileptic encephalopathy. The hope is that this will improve developmental outcome and reduce the morbidity and mortality associated with the syndrome. This has yet to be demonstrated and will require long-term longitudinal studies which we along with other groups are establishing.

The sodium channel mutation is implicated in all the comorbidities seen in this condition: the epileptic seizures, the intellectual disability, the dystonia, the ataxia, the encephalopathy and the behaviour problems.

The comorbidity of epilepsy and major psychiatric disorders has been much debated. In our studies of two Scottish families with a form of frontal lobe epilepsy called autosomal dominant nocturnal frontal lobe epilepsy (ADNFLE), we noted a high incidence of psychological disorders (McLellan et al. 2003). ADNFLE is caused by mutations in subunits of a neuronal nicotinic acetylcholine receptor which is a voltage-gated ion channel. In the families we studied we were uncertain whether the psychological problems such as anxiety disorders, depression and low self-esteem were non-specific consequences of delayed diagnosis of epilepsy and impact of epilepsy on quality of life or were part of a behavioural phenotype associated with the genetic mutation. Since then, three further papers have reported memory deficits, psychotic disorders, mood disorders and incapacitating apathy in families with ADNFLE (Magnusson et al. 2003, Bertrand et al. 2005, Derry et al. 2008). It is therefore highly likely that these symptoms are related to receptor function in the brain.

The neurological channelopathies are providing important insights into the pathogenesis of many of the comorbidities seen in clinical practice. This is an exciting field where the clinician, the molecular geneticist, the cell physiologist and the pharmacologist can all work together to translate clinical data into basic science advances which in turn will lead to better understanding of the disease and to new therapies.

REFERENCES

Berkovic SF, Harkin L, McMahon JM, et al. (2006) De-novo mutations of the sodium channel gene SCN1A in alleged vaccine encephalopathy: a retrospective study. *Lancet Neurol* **5**(6), 488–492.

Bertrand D, Elmslie F, Hughes E, et al. (2005) The CHRNB2 mutation I312M is associated with epilepsy and distinct memory deficits. *Neurobiol Dis* **20**, 799–804.

Biervert C, Schroeder BC, Kubisch C. et al. (1998) A potassium channel mutation in neonatal human epilepsy. *Science* **38**, 233–243.

Browne DL, Gancher ST, Nutt JG, et al. (1994) Episodic ataxia/myokymia syndrome is associated with point mutations in the human potassium channel gene, KCNA1. *Nat Genet* **8**, 136–140.

Cassé-Perrot C, Wolff M, Dravet C (2001) Neuropsychological effects of severe myoclonic epilepsy in infancy. In: Jambaqué I, Lassonde M, Dulac O (eds) *The Neuropsychology of Childhood Epilepsy*, New York: Plenum Press/Kluwer Academic, pp. 131–140.

Charlier C, Singh NA, Ryan SG (1998) A pore mutation in a novel KQT-like channel gene in an idiopathic epilepsy family. *Nat Genet* **18**, 53–55.

Chiron C, Marchand MC, Tran A, et al. (2000) Stiripentol in severe myoclonic epilepsy in infancy: a randomised placebo-controlled syndrome-dedicated trial. STICLO Study Group. *Lancet* **356**, 1638–1642.

Claes L, Del Favero J, Ceulemans B, Lagae L, van Broeckhoven C, de Jonghe P (2001) De novo mutations in the sodium channel gene SCN1A causes severe myoclonic epilepsy of infancy. *Am J Hum Genet* **68**, 1327–1332.

Depienne C, Trouillard O, Saint-Martin C, et al. (2008) Spectrum of SCN1A gene mutations associated with Dravet syndrome: analysis of 333 patients. *J Med Genet* **46**(3), 183–191.

Derry CP, Heron SE, Phillips F, et al. (2008) Severe autosomal dominant nocturnal frontal lobe epilepsy associated with psychiatric disorders and intellectual disability. *Epilepsia* **49**, 2125–2129.

Dravet C (1978) Les epilepsies graves de l'enfant. *Vie Med* **8**, 543–548.

Dravet C, Bureau M, Guerrini R, Giraud N, Roger J (1992) Severe myoclonic epilepsy in infants. In: Roger J, Bureau M, Dravet C, Dreiffuss FE, Perret A, Wolf P (eds) *Epileptic Syndromes in Infancy, Childhood and Adolescence*, 2nd edn. London: John Libbey, pp. 75–88.

Dravet C, Bureau M, Oguni H, Fukuyama Y, Cokar O (2002) Severe myoclonic epilepsy in infancy (Dravet Syndrome). In: Roger J, Bureau M, Dravet Ch, Genton P, Tassinari CA, Wolf P (eds) *Epileptic Syndromes in Infancy, Childhood and Adolescence*, 3rd edn. London: John Libbey, pp 81–103.

Eunson LH, Rear R, Zuberi SM, et al. (2000) Clinical, genetic and expression studies of mutations in the potassium channel gene KCNA1 reveal new phenotypic variability. *Ann Neurol* **48**, 647–656.

Fletcher CF, Frankel WN (1999) Ataxic mouse mutants and molecular mechanisms of absence epilepsy. *Hum Mol Genet* **8**, 1907–1912.

Fujiwara T, Sugawara T, Mazaki-Miyazaki E, et al. (2003) Mutations of sodium channel alpha subunit type 1 (SCN1A) in intractable childhood epilepsies with frequent generalised tonic-clonic seizures. *Brain* **126**, 531–546.

Griggs RC, Moxley RT 3rd, Lafrance RA, McQuillen J (1978) Hereditary paroxysmal ataxia: response to acetazolamide. *Neurology* **28**, 1259–1264.

Harkin LA, McMahon JM, Iona X, et al. (2007) The spectrum of SCN1A-related infantile epileptic encephalopathies. *Brain* **130**(Pt 3), 843–852.

Hille B (2001) *Ion Channels of Excitable Membranes*. Sunderland, MA: Sinauer Associates.

Hille B, Armstrong CM, Mackinnon R (1999) Ion channels: from idea to reality. *Nat Med* **5**, 1105–1109.

Hindocha N, Nashef L, Elmslie F, et al. (2008) Two cases of sudden unexpected death in epilepsy in a GEFS+ family with an SCN1A mutation. *Epilepsia* **49**(2), 360–365.

Hodgkin AL, Huxley AF (1952) Currents carried by sodium and potassium ions through the membrane of the giant axon of *Loligo*. *J Physiol* **116**, 449–472.

Imbrici P, Jaffe SL, Eunson LH, et al. (2004) Dysfunction of the brain calcium channel CaV2.1 in absence epilepsy and episodic ataxia. *Brain* **127**, 2682–2692.

Jen JC, Graves TD, Hess EJ, Hanna MG, Griggs RC, Baloh RW (2007) Primary episodic ataxias: diagnosis, pathogenesis and treatment. *Brain* 130, 2484–2493.

Jouvenceau A, Eunson LH, Spauschus A, et al. (2001) Human epilepsy associated with dysfunction of the brain P/Q-type calcium channel. *Lancet* **358**(9284), 801–807.

Kassai B, Chiron C, Augier, et al. (2008) Severe myoclonic epilepsy in infancy: a systematic review and a meta-analysis of individual patient data. *Epilepsia* **49**, 342–348.

Magnusson A, Stordal E, Brodtkorb E, Steinlein O (2003) Schizophrenia, psychotic illness and other psychiatric symptoms in families with autosomal dominant nocturnal frontal lobe epilepsy caused by different mutations. *Psychiatr Genet* **13**(2), 91–95.

McLellan A, Phillips HA, Rittey C, et al. (2003) Phenotypic comparison of two Scottish families with mutations in different genes causing autosomal dominant nocturnal frontal lobe epilepsy. *Epilepsia* **44**(4), 613–617.

Neher E, Sakman B (1976) Single channel currents recorded from membrane of denervated frog muscle fibres. *Nature* **260**, 799–802.

Ohki T, Watanabe K, Negoro K, et al. (1997) Severe myoclonic epilepsy in infancy: evolution of seizures. *Seizure* **6**, 219–224.

Ohtsuka Y, Ohmori I, Ogino T, Ouchida M, Shimizu K, Oka E (2003) Paroxysmal movement disorders in severe myoclonic epilepsy in infancy. *Brain Dev* **25**, 401–405.

Ophoff RA, Terwindt GM, Vergouwe MN, et al. (1996) Familial hemiplegic migraine and episodic ataxia type-2 are caused by mutations in the Ca2+ channel gene CACNL1A4. *Cell* **87**, 543–552.

Ragsdale DS (2008) How do mutant Nav1.1 sodium channels cause epilepsy? *Brain Res Rev* **58**, 149–159.

Vincent A, Buckley C, Schott JM, et al. (2004) Potassium channel antibody-associated encephalopathy: a potentially immunotherapy-responsive form of limbic encephalitis. *Brain* **127**, 701–712.

Wang Q, Curren ME, Splawski I, et al. (1996) Positional cloning of a novel potassium channel gene: KVLQT1 mutations cause cardiac arrhythmias. *Nat Genet* **12**, 17–23.

Zuberi SM (2003) Central nervous system/neuromuscular channelopathies. *Eur J Paediatr Neurol* **7**, 187–190.

Zuberi SM, Eunson LH, Spauschus A, et al. (1999) A novel mutation in the human voltage-gated potassium channel gene (Kv1.1) associates with episodic ataxia type 1 and sometimes with partial epilepsy. *Brain* **122**, 817–825.

9
INCREASED LONGEVITY AND THE COMORBIDITIES ASSOCIATED WITH INTELLECTUAL AND DEVELOPMENTAL DISABILITY

Alan H Bittles and Emma J Glasson

The health and survival of people with intellectual and developmental disabilities (IDD) have increased significantly during the past century, aided by deinstitutionalisation and improved access to health care. In high-income countries, life expectancy estimates are now approximately 70 years for people with mild IDD and 60 years for those with more severe levels of IDD. The increasing survival of people with IDD will result in a greater risk of age-related morbidity, and both adult-onset cancers and non-malignant disorders, especially since age-related comorbidities generally appear at younger ages than in the general population. In disorders such as Down syndrome, a 'whole of life' approach to health care is required, with greater focus especially needed during the period spanning middle age to senescence so that appropriate management regimes can be implemented on an individual and disorder-specific basis. Secondary conditions that arise later in adulthood, including osteoporosis, obesity, cardiovascular disease, epilepsy and dementia, additionally need to be considered within health care plans. The types of interventions offered and continuity of care are of critical importance, especially since people with IDD, including those with Down syndrome, will frequently outlive their parents and even their siblings.

Approximately 1–4% of people in developed countries exhibit some degree of intellectual and developmental disability (IDD) (Roeleveld et al. 1997, WHO 2001, Australian Institute of Health and Welfare 2003), and an estimated 0.5–1.0% of the population require daily support because of IDD (Australian Institute of Health and Welfare 2003). The exact population prevalence of IDD is difficult to determine, as screening studies only provide a measure of prevalence at a particular point in time. Additional problems arise in ascertainment, since people with IDD are at risk of premature mortality, young children are difficult to assess, and through time older children or adults who score poorly on IQ assessments may have acquired adaptive behaviour skills which place them outside the definitions of IDD (Australian Institute of Health and Welfare 2003).

Intellectual and developmental disabilities are determined by performance in cognition (IQ) and adaptive behaviour (life skills) assessments. A diagnosis is given when scores on both instruments fall at least two standard deviations below the mean of 100 points (i.e. achieving less than 70 points). The degree of disability is described by the distance of scores from the mean, usually expressed by three levels of disability. People with a mild level of disability (i.e. with scores ranging from approximately 55 to 69) form the largest subgroup and represent some 85% of the total population with IDD. By comparison, about 10% of cases have moderate disability (a score between 40 and 54) and 5% have severe disability (a score less than 40 points) (American Psychiatric Association 1994).

INCREASED LIFE EXPECTANCY OF PEOPLE WITH INTELLECTUAL AND DEVELOPMENTAL DISABILITIES

The health of people in high-income countries improved significantly during the 20th century, due to advances in medicine, improved health care resources and treatments, and the overall improvements in lifestyle, housing and nutrition that accompanied economic growth. As a result, in Australia, infant mortality (deaths to one year of age) decreased from 107 per 1000 to 5 per 1000 births between 1902 and 2002 (Australian Bureau of Statistics 2004), and overall life expectancy rose from 55 to 76 years for males and 59 to 82 years for females (Australian Bureau of Statistics 2002), with further increases to 79 years for males and 84 years for females by 2006 (Australian Bureau of Statistics 2008). The health care and survival of people with IDD also increased, although from a much lower starting level and commencing at a later date. Nevertheless, by the end of the 20th century in North America, Western Europe and Oceania, survival estimates were approximately 70 years of age for people with mild IDD and 60 years for those with severe levels of IDD (Janicki et al. 1999, Patja et al. 2000, Bittles et al. 2002). For milder forms of IDD, life expectancies are almost comparable to those in the general population (Patja et al. 2000).

DEINSTITUTIONALISATION

During the mid-20th century many large North American and Western European institutions providing living accommodation and care for people with IDD experienced severe overcrowding, understaffing and limitations on their allocated resources. These problems were exacerbated by reports of the inhumane treatment of residents, who often lacked stimulation, interaction or even basic health and social care (Nirje 1969a). In addition, the health of residents frequently was impaired by outbreaks of infectious respiratory diseases (Polednak 1977) and *Helicobacter pylori* infection was common (Duff et al. 2001, Wallace et al. 2002).

The large institutions offering long-term accommodation were eventually closed during the latter half of the century, accompanied by a positive shift in general attitudes among health professionals towards people with IDD and improved overall access to treatment. Many of these changes were based on the Scandinavian 'normalisation principle', which advocated matching of the everyday living conditions of people with IDD with those of mainstream society (Nirje 1969b). This led to the establishment of smaller, better resourced centres with trained health care workers and specialised support structures to facilitate care needs, and encouragement for people with IDD to live with their family for as long as possible (Dybwad 1969).

Public attitudes towards IDD also changed, with greater acceptance that adults with disabilities should be enabled to live independently in the community, and support for their integration into the education sector and the workforce. These changes have resulted in increased opportunities for people with IDD to contribute to society through independent and partially dependent social, sporting and economic roles (Carek et al. 2002). Greatly improved access to general health care, management and interventions has followed, although the provision of appropriate services for this vulnerable section of the population is still inconsistent in many countries (Mencap 1998, WHO 2000, Hogg et al. 2001, US Public Health Service 2001).

Comorbidities associated with intellectual and developmental disabilities

Individuals with IDD differ widely in the aetiology of their IDD, clinical profile and degree of impairment, resulting in diverse patterns of comorbidities and required levels of intervention and support needs. The care of individuals with IDD is therefore complex, especially since health concerns may be compounded by communication difficulties and dependence on others for monitoring and responding to their needs. For these reasons, and despite a higher prevalence of medical problems, people with IDD may be less likely to participate in screening programmes or to undergo regular medical checks (Sullivan et al. 2003, Owens et al. 2006). Thus improved education and awareness are needed among the professional community and carers to monitor comorbidities that are expected to arise over time, with specific disorders manifesting at certain ages in particular syndromes (WHO 2000).

Sensory impairment often accompanies advancing age and if left untreated it can complicate the diagnosis and management of other health problems. Visual impairment, particularly associated with strabismus and refractive errors, is significantly more common among people with IDD than in the general population (Carvill 2001), and it is positively correlated with advancing age and increased severity of symptoms (Owens et al. 2006). A study conducted in The Netherlands indicated that visual impairment affected 2.2% of young adults with mild IDD not due to Down syndrome, and 66.7% of older persons with profound IDD and Down syndrome (van Splunder et al. 2006). In these two subgroups the overall prevalence of blindness ranged from 0.7% to 38.9% (van Splunder et al. 2006).

Hearing loss is 40–100 times more common than in the general population (Carvill 2001) and it is associated with risk factors that include congenital defects (such as the presence of craniofacial syndromes), obstetric events (including intrauterine infections) and late-onset occurrences (such as meningitis) (Evenhuis 1996). Conductive hearing loss or impacted wax accretion is prevalent in both institutionalised and community-based groups, and may remain undiagnosed or underestimated without regular testing (Evenhuis 1996, Carvill 2001, Kerr et al. 2003). The combination of hearing and visual impairments is more common after 50 years of age, with 3% of those less than 50 years and 11% of those over 50 years being affected in one cross-sectional study (Meuwese-Jongejeugd et al. 2008). In addition to age, the presence of these dual sensory impairments was also positively correlated with severity of disability and a diagnosis of Down syndrome.

Poor oral health (Owens et al. 2006), obesity (Rimmer & Yamaki 2006), cardiovascular disease (van den Akker et al. 2006) and dementia (Janicki & Dalton 2000) are typical examples of the secondary conditions that may increase in prevalence during adulthood. Osteoporosis may also develop, especially in individuals with restricted mobility or in association with anticonvulsant medications (Jaffe et al. 2005).

The prevalence and persistence of psychopathologies comorbid with IDD in children and young adults have been demonstrated in an extended Australian study of urban and rural populations (Einfeld et al. 2006). People with IDD are generally at higher risk of schizophrenia, depression, maladaptive disorders, pervasive developmental disorders and behavioural abnormalities, including aggression or self-injury. Major psychotic disorders, such as depression or schizophrenia, have been identified in up to 15% of all people with IDD (Gustavson et al. 2005, Stromme & Diseth 2000). Psychiatric morbidity, including emotional and/or behavioural symptomatology, is more prevalent with IDD and affects approximately 40% of cases, i.e. occurring at approximately three times the reported rate in the general population (Emerson 2003, Cooper et al. 2007).

These comorbid disorders commonly occur as part of the phenotype of specific syndromes which cause IDD and, for example, Down syndrome is frequently comorbid with Alzheimer disease (Mann 1988, Prasher et al. 1997), with depression also commonly observed in such cases (McCarron et al. 2005). Autistic symptoms often are reported in people with fragile X syndrome (Hatton et al. 2006), and eating disorders, self-injury and obsessive compulsive disorders are common among those with Prader–Willi syndrome (Dykens et al. 1996, Hartley et al. 2005, Thomson et al. 2006). Sensory impairments, epilepsy and brain trauma have also been associated with increased risk of psychiatric illness, consequently increasing support requirements and overall carer burden.

AGEING

In overall terms, the age-related comorbidities experienced by people with IDD appear at younger ages than in the general population and may progress rapidly in a poorly managed environment, particularly if the problems are neglected or inadequately communicated to carers. Polypharmacy issues may arise, especially in community settings (Lott et al. 2004), which can result in serious behavioural side-effects and be potentially life-threatening if not appropriately monitored (WHO 2000, Huber et al. 2008).

The functional abilities of people with IDD often appear to improve later in life, mainly because of early mortality among those with more severe degrees of disability who have shorter lifespans (Holland 2000). However, there are many conditions which arise later in adulthood that need particular attention and support. These include higher frequencies of already at-risk disorders, such as epilepsy, dementia and osteoporosis. Because of their lower peak bone mass and a loss of peak mass after menopause, females in the general population have a greater probability of developing osteoporosis, with high fracture risk after 70 years of age (Schrager 2006). In the presence of reduced mobility and/or prescription of long-term anticonvulsants, many women with IDD exhibit an increased risk of reduced bone density and bone fractures at a comparatively earlier age (Schrager 2006). Other age-related disorders, such as obesity and cardiovascular disease, are significantly affected by both lifestyle and biological predisposition.

Psychological and social life stages that typically characterize adulthood in the general community are often poorly researched among the IDD population. Improved education and advice are needed on sexuality issues, including menopause, accompanied by research into the precise changes in hormone levels and ovarian function for women with different syndromes and comorbidities (WHO 2000). In many countries, parenthood is regarded as an emerging right for people with IDD, but the situation is complex given the levels of support that may be required (Kandel et al. 2005). Substantial ethical and quality of life issues can be anticipated in assisting older people with IDD to attain optimal control of their lives. Examples include the potential role of people with IDD as organ recipients or donors, access to medical procedures and priorities on waiting lists, and the provision of informed consent for treatment (Savulescu 2001, Martens et al. 2006).

Problems surrounding irregular employment and retirement require further exploration (Ashman et al. 1995), because of the associations with decreased quality of life and psychological conditions, such as depression or boredom, that can occur in response to these life stages (Rogers et al. 1998, Esbensen & Benson 2006). If not adequately addressed, poorly managed social needs may impact adversely on general health, and loneliness and depression are significant risks for older people with IDD, who may lose existing friends and fail to develop new friendships, or whose limited social networks may generate excessive unstructured free time (Duvdevany & Arar 2004). Behavioural disturbance and emotional distress similarly may go unrecognised when people with IDD lose a parent, but could be addressed with bereavement counselling and coping strategies that previously have shown measurable benefits (Dowling et al. 2006). Comprehensive research into issues associated with pain expression and palliative care is merited (Oberlander & Symons 2006), including investigations into direct patient experiences and their comprehension of issues surrounding death, as well as support mechanisms and appropriate management at the end of life phase (Tuffrey-Wijne 2003).

Down syndrome

Down syndrome is arguably the best known genetic cause of IDD and the disorder has been extensively investigated since its original description by Dr James Langdon Down in 1866. Down believed that the form of 'mongolian idiocy' that now bears his name was caused by degeneracy resulting from parental tuberculosis (Down 1866). No such correlation has been demonstrated and other environmental factors claimed to have resulted in localised clusters of Down syndrome have similarly been discounted, for example, post-Chernobyl radio-active contamination in Germany (Burkart et al. 1997) and radio-active fall-out from a UK nuclear plant affecting the east coast of Ireland (Dean et al. 2000).

There is a strong positive association with advanced maternal age, and among women aged 35 years and older the mean birth prevalence of Down syndrome has been estimated at 1 per 338 live births, with an increase to 1 per 32 live births by 45 years of age (Morris et al. 2005). An association between consanguineous marriage and Down syndrome was reported in a number of studies, with the suggestion that there may be an autosomal gene(s) that controls mitotic non-disjunction (Alfi et al. 1980, Farag & Teebi 1988, Roberts et al. 1991, de Braekeleer et al. 1994). However, since other researchers were unable to substantiate this

TABLE 9.1
Down syndrome livebirths, pregnancy terminations and stillbirths per 1000 births in Western Australia, 1980–2004

	1980	1985	1990	1995	2000	2004
Livebirths	1.1	1.2	1.1	1.1	1.3	1.1
Termination of pregnancy	0.0	0.3	0.3	1.1	1.7	1.7
Stillbirths	0.0	0.0	0.1	0.0	0.1	0.1
All Down syndrome pregnancies	1.1	1.5	1.6	2.2	3.1	2.9

Source: Bittles et al. 2007.

claim (Devoto et al. 1985, Hamamy et al. 1990, Başaran et al. 1992, Cereijo & Martínez Frías 1993), no consistent association seems likely across populations.

FROM BIRTH TO ADULTHOOD

Down syndrome accounts for 12–15% of cases of IDD (Wellesley et al. 1991, Alessandri et al. 1996, Hou et al. 1998, Bittles et al. 2002), and the disorder occurs in 1 per 650 to 1 per 1000 live births (Baird & Sadovnick 1987, Stoll et al. 1998, Frid et al. 1999). Globally, it has been estimated that around 217,000 infants with Down syndrome are born per year (March of Dimes 2006), with approximately 95% of all cases of Down syndrome due to trisomy 21 and the remainder associated with autosomal translocations or mosaicism. The extra chromosome is of maternal origin in 85% of cases of trisomy 21, most commonly (80%) caused by non-disjunction at the first meiotic division. While dosage-sensitive genes contained in a critical segment of chromosome 21 appear to be involved in the characteristic disease phenotype, trisomy alone is not sufficient to produce the types of hippocampal impairment typically seen in Down syndrome (Olson et al. 2004, 2007).

Despite the availability of prenatal testing and the option of termination of Down syndrome pregnancies, the number of Down syndrome live births has remained relatively constant over the last generation, primarily due to a widespread increase in mean maternal age (Binkert et al. 2002, Nicholson & Alberman 1992, O'Leary et al. 1996), and in some countries the birth incidence has increased (Metneki & Czeizel 2005, Crane & Morris 2006). This situation is illustrated in Table 9.1, based on data collected in Western Australia from 1980 to 2004, where pregnancies among women aged 35 years or above increased from 4.8% in 1980 to 18.6% in 2004. The average number of terminations of Down syndrome pregnancies rose each decade from 18% per year (1980–1989) to 42% (1990–1999), and then to 60% of pregnancies (2000–2004). Therefore between 1980 and 2004 the greater annual numbers of Down syndrome pregnancies were effectively balanced by increasing pregnancy terminations, resulting in similar proportions of people born with Down syndrome across the study period (Bittles et al. 2007).

In Western countries, Down syndrome provides an instructive example of improved survival in response to better health care opportunities, with an increase in life expectancy of just under one year of age for each calendar year since the 1950s (Bittles & Glasson 2004). This has meant an increase in the mean life expectancy of people with Down syndrome from 12 years of age in 1949 (Penrose 1949) to approximately 60 years of age by 2000 (Bittles & Glasson 2004). Survival in infancy and childhood also has improved markedly. Thus, while an infant born with Down syndrome in the mid-20th century had only a 45% chance of surviving to one year (Record & Smith 1955), survival had increased to 96% by the last decade of the century, particularly if a heart defect was absent or could be repaired early in life (Bell et al. 1989, Hayes et al. 1997, Masuda et al. 2005). Despite these improvements, problems remain with respect to low birthweight babies with Down syndrome. Children with Down syndrome also have higher death rates from sepsis (Garrison et al. 2005), and major ethnic disparities in survival are still apparent (Leonard et al. 2000, Day et al. 2005, Rasmussen et al. 2006).

Down syndrome is associated with elevated levels of cardiac, gastrointestinal, immunological, respiratory, sensory and orthopaedic problems at birth (Pueschel et al. 1995, van Allen et al. 1999), and there is growth impairment in childhood (Myrelid et al. 2002). Congenital heart defects have been reported in 42–60% of children with Down syndrome (Tubman et al. 1991, Wells et al. 1994, Venugopalan & Agarwal 2003, Vida et al. 2005), and the disorder is a causative factor in approximately 10% of all children identified with a congenital cardiac anomaly (Eskedal et al. 2004). Significant interpopulation differences have been reported in the specific types of congenital heart defect detected (Lo et al. 1989, Tubman et al. 1991, Wells et al. 1994, Vida et al. 2005), and additional cardiac problems may arise in populations with high rates of consanguineous marriage (Venugopalan & Agarwal 2003).

Spontaneous closure of ventricular defects has been reported in a substantial number of people with Down syndrome (Dunlop et al. 2004). Where surgery was undertaken to correct a congenital heart defect, studies from a wide range of countries indicate that patients with Down syndrome had similar or even superior survival outcomes to children with normal chromosomal karyotypes (Reller & Morris 1998, Al-Hay et al. 2003, Dunlop et al. 2004, Formigari et al. 2004, Frid et al. 2004, Masuda et al. 2005, Roussot et al. 2006). However, there also is evidence that children with Down syndrome undergoing surgery for non-cardiac procedures are more likely to experience anaesthesia-related complications, including brachycardia, natural airway obstruction and postintubation croup (Borland et al. 2004).

Childhood leukaemia, both acute lymphoblastic and acute non-lymphoblastic, is the most characteristic early malignancy in Down syndrome, with an incidence over 20 times higher than the comparable general population (Fong & Brodeur 1987, Hasle et al. 2000, Chessells et al. 2001, Hogg et al. 2001, Hill et al. 2003, Goldacre et al. 2004, Sullivan et al. 2007). By comparison, lower rates of neuroblastoma and nephroblastoma have been found in children with Down syndrome (Satgé et al. 1998).

The improved survival rates of children and young adults with Down syndrome, combined with better investigative techniques and levels of health care, have resulted in an increasingly wide range of comorbid genetic anomalies being diagnosed. In Ireland 15% of patients with Hirschsprung disease had Down syndrome (Menezes & Puri 2005) and in other countries patients with Down syndrome and β-thalassaemia (Keser et al. 2001), and

Down syndrome with type 1 neurofibromatosis and breast cancer (Satgé et al. 2004) also have been reported. Given these examples, it seems prudent to assume that further examples of otherwise uncommon disease concurrences will be found if more rigorous investigative procedures are routinely adopted in patients with Down syndrome.

AGEING

Many of the current cohorts of people with Down syndrome in high-income countries are expected to live to over 60 years of age, especially individuals who do not have congenital heart disorders (Janicki et al. 1999, Glasson et al. 2002). Males in Australia with Down syndrome had an approximately three year higher mean life expectancy than females (Glasson et al. 2003). This does not appear to be the case in The Netherlands (Coppus et al. 2008a), although as noted by the authors, there was a disproportionate number of males in their middle-aged study cohort, which may be indicative of greater female mortality at younger ages. The increased prevalence of people with Down syndrome and their predicted survival to more advanced ages will inevitably result in greater numbers living in the community, with increased demands for specialist care given the particular patterns of comorbidity that are expected to appear at certain life stages. In adulthood, pneumonia and other respiratory infections are the most common causes of death, with coronary artery disease, cardiac, renal and respiratory failure, cerebrovascular accident and cancers additional important disorders (Bittles et al. 2007).

The physical manifestations of ageing among people with Down syndrome may begin some 30 years earlier than in the general population (Holland 2000). Epilepsy increases steadily in prevalence with advancing age, affecting some 30% of patients over 60 years of age (Pueschel et al. 1995, van Allen et al. 1999, Puri et al. 2001, McDermott et al. 2005). Among individuals with Down syndrome, late-onset epilepsy is associated with Alzheimer disease whereas dementia is generally absent among those with early-onset epilepsy (Menéndez 2005).

As previously noted, visual and hearing impairments significantly increase with age from the elevated rates which initially place children with Down syndrome at greater risk than children with other forms of IDD (Owens et al. 2006), and they may cause additional concerns if not treated. Adult obesity, mainly affecting females rather than males, is more commonly associated with Down syndrome than many other syndromes associated with IDD (Melville et al. 2005, Rimmer & Yamaki 2006), and may contribute to the spinal problems that have been observed in individuals with Down syndrome and scoliosis (Milbrandt & Johnston 2005).

Increased rates of testicular, pancreatic, ovarian and uterine cancers, skin cancers, retinoblastoma and malignant tumours of the brain all have been reported (Satgé et al. 1998, Hasle et al. 2000, Patja et al. 2001), with higher risks of brain and stomach cancers in males, and corpus uteri and colorectal cancer in females (Sullivan et al. 2004). Occasional cases of other rare malignancies, such as Waldenstrom macroglobinaemia, have been observed (Sullivan et al. 2007), and the elevated prevalence of *H. pylori* infections in institutionalised persons may be responsible for a higher incidence of the premalignant Barrett oesophagus (Bohmer et al. 1997).

A number of publications have drawn attention to the lower rates of breast cancer among women with Down syndrome of reproductive and postreproductive age (Hasle et al. 2000, Satgé et al. 2001, Satgé & Sasco 2002), and it has been suggested that the cellular micro-environment in Down syndrome may exert an inhibitory effect on tumour proliferation via altered angiogenesis (Bénard et al. 2005). Unfortunately, it also has been shown that, in general terms, women with Down syndrome and other forms of IDD are less likely to receive breast screening and so be diagnosed with breast cancer (Piachaud & Rohde 1998, Sullivan et al. 2003). As women with all forms of IDD are surviving to ages where the incidence of breast cancer increases sharply, the implementation of good practice guidelines for breast and cervical cancer screening is therefore of increasing importance (National Health Service Cancer Screening Programme 2000, Satgé & Sasco 2002).

Abnormal thyroid dysfunction, usually decreased function, has been reported in up to a third of adults with Down syndrome (Prasher & Haque 2005). Since low thyroid function can occur in otherwise healthy patients with Down syndrome, it is unclear whether it is a characteristic feature of the syndrome or simply represents a consequence of premature ageing (Prasher & Haque 2005). In either case, the use of Down syndrome-specific charts for normal thyroid function would appear appropriate, comparable to those used for the assessment of height which typically is reduced in affected adults (Toledo et al. 1999).

Clinical symptoms associated with Alzheimer disease and other neuropathological features, such as memory loss and cognitive decline, may not be present at the time of death, although they are more common in people with Down syndrome over the age of 55 years (Lai et al. 1989, Dalton & Wisniewski 1990, Visser et al. 1997, Zigman et al. 1997, Coppus et al. 2006, 2008a). Due to difficulties in diagnosis, there is considerable uncertainty as to the age at onset of Alzheimer disease in people with Down syndrome. Autopsy evidence suggests that the characteristic neuropathological features of Alzheimer disease are present in about 8% of people in their second decade, increasing to 80% by the fourth decade of life (Mann 1988), and over 80% of persons with Down syndrome and dementia develop seizures (Menéndez 2005).

It has been proposed that the excess risk of Alzheimer disease may be due to an extra copy of the amyloid precursor protein (APP) gene located on chromosome 21. However, as in the general population, it also has been shown that the apolipoprotein ε4 (APOE4) allele is an independent risk factor adversely influencing the frequency and manifestations of dementia in people with Down syndrome (Deb et al. 2000), including their social competence scores (Coppus et al. 2008b). There also is a substantially higher amyloid burden in individuals who inherit APOE4, present even in children and adolescents with Down syndrome (Mehta et al. 2007), which in part could explain the greater prevalence of Alzheimer disease in people with the disorder (Hyman et al. 1995, Coppus et al. 2008b).

Projected health trends

Better prevention methods and medical interventions assisted by improved knowledge, education and access to treatments should result in a decrease in the prevalence of at least some of the comorbid conditions associated with IDD. At the same time, a number of disorders, including Down syndrome, remain relatively common and other conditions, such as autism, continue to increase in community prevalence due to better ascertainment and more efficient diagnostic procedures (Fombonne et al. 2006). Improved care and interventions have enhanced overall community health and so more people, including those with IDD, are living longer, albeit with increased risks of morbidity.

FUTURE NEEDS

Deinstitutionalisation has led to people with IDD following an independent or partially independent lifestyle within the community, using the same health care pathways and facilities as the general population. While progress in this area is welcome, several potential disadvantages need to be addressed, in particular the possibility that access to trained and experienced health professionals has diminished and regular health checks may not be efficiently regulated (Nottestad & Linaker 1999, Dovey & Webb 2000). Because of the subtle and specialist problems which can arise in people with IDD, general medical practitioners may have difficulties in terms of the necessary experience and skills to ensure optimum diagnosis and treatment, for example, in the monitoring of visual problems (Kerr et al. 2003). In overall terms, GPs treating patients with IDD are faced with a greater workload, with 1.7 times more visits recorded per person in a recent Dutch study (Straetmans et al. 2007). Improved training opportunities for primary health care professionals (Melville et al. 2006) and the introduction of health screening programmes (Cooper et al. 2006) could help to ease this burden.

Community-based living is often associated with less structured regimes and hence greater exposure to suboptimal lifestyle choices. Under such circumstances, lifestyle diseases, such as obesity, diabetes, blood pressure anomalies and cardiovascular illness, are more likely to develop, and individuals are more prone to engage in risk-taking behaviour, including smoking and substance abuse. People with Down syndrome exhibit higher social competencies by comparison with disorders such as Prader–Willi or Williams syndrome (Rosner et al. 2004). Nevertheless, an interview-based study of health knowledge and behaviour conducted on adolescents with Down syndrome and their families found that the adolescents had insufficient levels of understanding to enable them to live independently (Jobling & Cuskelly 2006).

More generally, research on the prevalence of obesity in people with IDD has shown that the lowest rates occurred among individuals resident in institutions, with a higher percentage in community-based residential homes, and the highest levels among those living with family members (Rimmer & Yamaki 2006). These findings suggest that monitoring the multifactorial antecedents of obesity and other health-related issues, and the complexity of both general and acute care, may be a problem among relatives caring for people with IDD in the family home setting.

Greater focus is needed on disorders that emerge during middle age to senescence so that appropriate management regimes can be implemented, with more detailed studies required to determine whether particular syndromes are prone to specific age-related problems and the influence of factors such as diet and exercise on these emergent problems. To encourage such investigations, the World Health Organization has recommended that health care providers adopt a total lifespan approach which recognises the progression of specific diseases and the need for appropriate therapeutic interventions (WHO 2000).

Initiatives of this type are quite costly and it has been estimated that at least 9.0% of disease-specific health care costs in The Netherlands are devoted to the needs of people with IDD, with age-related peaks in treatment costs during the 25–45 year range for both males and females, and over 70 years of age due to dementia, particularly among females (Polder et al. 2002). Using data from multiple surveys and reports, the lifetime costs for people with IDD in the USA born during the year 2000 were estimated to total US$51.2 billion, of which approximately US$12 billion was attributed to direct costs (Centers for Disease Control 2004). The Dutch and US data therefore support the need for more efficient prevention programmes to reduce the population prevalence of causes of IDD, which led the American College of Obstetricians and Gynecologists to recommend that all pregnancies in the USA be screened for Down syndrome (American College of Obstetricians and Gyne-cologists 2007). The proposal was, however, criticised by the National Down Syndrome Society, with counter-recommendations that expectant mothers should not be unduly influ-enced either to undergo prenatal testing for the condition or to terminate a pregnancy in the event of a positive diagnosis (National Down Syndrome Society 2007).

The need for effective interventions in the primary care of people with IDD is incon-trovertible and should both benefit the health and well-being of affected individuals and help to constrain health expenditure. In addition, research is required to identify how indirect costs, such as social and community supports that enable people with IDD to live produc-tively within the community, might be reduced while maintaining a high quality of life. At the same time, complementary measures to assist the carers of persons with IDD and reduce the high levels of stress to which they may be subjected (Epel et al. 2004) are also essential, especially as these people themselves grow older (Glasson & Bittles 2008).

The collection, sharing and judicious application of comprehensive morbidity informa-tion for the middle and later years of life should greatly help in the process of informed decision making in all such cases. Electronic linkage of health data derived from different statutory bodies has resulted in demonstrable benefits for the IDD population in Western countries (Glasson & Hussain 2008). Continuation and expansion of this approach should enable a more precise and timely response to the many problems faced in providing the levels of care and support required by this burgeoning section of the global population.

REFERENCES

Alessandri L, Leonard H, Blum L, Bower C (1996) *Disability Counts. A Profile of Disability in Western Australia*. Perth, Western Australia: Disability Services Commission.

Alfi OS, Chang R, Azen SP (1980) Evidence for genetic control of nondisjunction in man. *Am J Hum Genet* **32**, 477–483.

Al-Hay AA, MacNeill SJ, Yacoub M, Shore DF, Shinebourne EA (2003) Complete atrioventricular septal defect, Down syndrome, and surgical outcome, risk factors. *Ann Thorac Surg* **75**, 412–421.

American College of Obstetricians and Gynecologists (2007) Practice Bulletin No. 77. Screening for fetal chromosomal abnormalities. *Obstet Gynecol* **109**, 217–227.

American Psychiatric Association (1994) *Diagnostic and Statistical Manual of Mental Disorders*. Washington, DC: American Psychiatric Association.

Ashman AF, Suttie JN, Bramley J (1995) Employment, retirement and elderly persons with an intellectual disability. *J Intellect Disabil Res* **39**, 107–115.

Australian Bureau of Statistics (2002) *Year Book Australia, 2002*. Canberra: Australian Bureau of Statistics.

Australian Bureau of Statistics (2004) *Health of Children, 2004*. Canberra: Australian Bureau of Statistics.

Australian Bureau of Statistics (2008) *Deaths, Australia, 2007*. Canberra: Australian Bureau of Statistics.

Australian Institute of Health and Welfare (2003) *Disability Prevalence and Trends*. Disability Series. Canberra: Australian Institute of Health and Welfare.

Baird PA, Sadovnick AD (1987) Life expectancy in Down syndrome. *J Pediatr* **110**, 849–854.

Başaran N, Cenani A, Şayli BS, et al. (1992) Consanguineous marriages among parents of Down patients. *Clin Genet* **42**, 13–15.

Bell JA, Pearn JH, Firman D (1989) Childhood deaths in Down's syndrome. Survival curves and causes of death from a total population study in Queensland, Australia, 1976 to 1985. *J Med Genet* **26**, 764–768.

Bénard J, Béron-Gaillard N, Satgé D (2005) Down's syndrome protects against breast cancer. Is a constitutional cell microenvironment the key? *Int J Cancer* **113**, 168–170.

Binkert F, Mutter M, Schinzel A (2002) Impact of prenatal diagnosis on the prevalence of live births with Down syndrome in the eastern half of Switzerland 1980–1996. *Swiss Med Wkly* **132**, 478–484.

Bittles AH, Glasson EJ (2004) Clinical, social and ethical implications of changing life expectancy in Down syndrome. *Dev Med Child Neurol* **46**, 282–286.

Bittles AH, Petterson BA, Sullivan SG, Hussain R, Glasson EJ, Montgomery PD (2002) The influence of intellectual disability on life expectancy. *J Gerontol A, Biol Sci Med Sci* **57**, M470-M472.

Bittles AH, Bower C, Hussain R, Glasson EJ (2007) The four ages of Down syndrome. *Eur J Public Health* **17**, 221–225

Bohmer CJ, Klinkenberg-Knol EC, Niezen-de Boer RC, Meuwissen SG (1997) The age-related incidences of oesophageal carcinoma in intellectually disabled individuals in institutes in The Netherlands. *Eur J Gastroenterol Hepatol* **9**, 589–592.

Borland LM, Colligan J, Brandom BW (2004) Frequency of anesthesia-related complications in children with Down syndrome under general anesthesia for noncardiac procedures. *Paediatr Anaesth* **14**, 733–738.

Burkart W, Grosche B, Schoetzau A (1997) Down syndrome clusters in Germany after the Chernobyl accident. *Radiat Res* **147**, 321–328.

Carek PJ, Dickerson LM, Hawkins A (2002) Special olympics, special athletes, special needs? *J S Carolina Med Assoc* **98**, 183–186.

Carvill S (2001) Sensory impairments, intellectual disability and psychiatry. *J Intellect Disabil Res* **45**, 467–483.

Centers for Disease Control (2004) Economic costs associated with mental retardation, cerebral palsy, hearing loss, and vision impairment – United States, 2003. *Morb Mortal Wkly Rep* **53**, 57–59.

Cereijo AI, Martínez-Frías ML (1993) Consanguineous marriages among parents of patients with Down syndrome. *Clin Genet* **44**, 221–222.

Chessells JM, Harrison G, Richards SM, et al. (2001) Down's syndrome and acute lymphoblastic leukaemia, clinical features and response to treatment. *Arch Dis Child* **85**, 321–325.

Cooper SA, Morrison J, Melville C, et al. (2006) Improving the health of people with intellectual disabilities, outcomes of a health screening programme after 1 year. *J Intellect Disabil Res* **50**, 667–677.

Cooper SA, Smiley E, Morrison J, Williamson A, Allan L (2007) Mental ill-health in adults with intellectual disabilities, prevalence and associated factors. *Br J Psychiatry* **190**, 27–35.

Coppus A, Evenhuis H, Verberne GJ, et al. (2006) Dementia and mortality in persons with Down's syndrome. *J Intellect Disabil Res* **50**, 768–777.

Coppus AM, Evenhuis HM, Verberne GJ, et al. (2008a) Survival in elderly persons with Down syndrome. *J Am Geriatr Soc* **56**, 2311–2316.

Coppus AM, Evenhuis HM, Verberne GJ, et al. (2008b) The impact of apolipoprotein E on dementia in persons with Down's syndrome. *Neurobiol Aging* **29**, 828–835.

Crane E, Morris JK (2006) Changes in maternal age in England and Wales – implications for Down syndrome. *Down's Syndr Res Pract* **10**, 41–43.

Dalton AJ, Wisniewski HM (1990) Down's syndrome and the dementia of Alzheimer's disease. *Int Rev Psychiatry* **2**, 43–52.

Day SM, Strauss DJ, Shavelle RM, Reynolds RJ (2005) Mortality and causes of death in persons with Down syndrome in California. *Dev Med Child Neurol* **47**, 171–176.

de Braekeleer M, Landry T, Cholette A (1994) Consanguinity and kinship in Down syndrome in Saguenay Lac-Saint-Jean (Québec). *Annal Génét* **37**, 86–88.

Dean G, Nevin NC, Mikkelsen M, et al. (2000) Investigation of a cluster of children with Down's syndrome born to mothers who had attended a school in Dundalk, Ireland. *Occup Environ Med* **57**, 793–804.

Deb S, Braganza J, Norton N, et al. (2000) APOE epsilon 4 influences the manifestation of Alzheimer's disease in adults with Down's syndrome. *Br J Psychiatry* **176**, 468–472.

Devoto M, Prosperi L, Bricarelli FD, et al. (1985) Frequency of consanguineous marriages among parents and grandparents of Down patients. *Hum Genet* **70**, 256–258.

Dovey S, Webb OJ (2000) General practitioners' perception of their role in care for people with intellectual disability. *J Intellect Disabil Res* **44**, 553–561.

Dowling S, Hubert J, White S, Hollins S (2006) Bereaved adults with intellectual disabilities, a combined randomized controlled trial and qualitative study of two community-based interventions. *J Intellect Disabil Res* **50**, 277–287.

Down JLH (1866) Observations on an ethnic classification of idiots. *London Hosp Rep 3* **S**, 259–262.

Duff M, Scheepers M, Cooper M, Hoghton M, Baddeley P (2001) *Helicobacter pylori*, has the killer escaped from the institution? A possible cause of increased stomach cancer in a population with intellectual disability. *J Intellect Disabil Res* **45**, 219–225.

Dunlop KA, Mulholland HC, Casey FA, Craig B, Gladstone DJ (2004) A ten year review of atrioventricular septal defects. *Cardiol Young* **14**, 15–23.

Duvdevany I, Arar E (2004) Leisure activities, friendships, and quality of life of persons with intellectual disability, foster homes vs community residential settings. *Int J Rehab Res* **27**, 289–296.

Dybwad G (1969) Action implications, USA today. In: Kugel RB, Wolfensberger W (eds) *Changing Patterns in Residential Services for the Mentally Retarded*. Washington, DC: President's Committee on Mental Retardation, pp. 383–428.

Dykens EM, Leckman JF, Cassidy SB (1996) Obsessions and compulsions in Prader–Willi syndrome. *J Child Psychol Psychiatr* **37**, 995–1002.

Einfeld SL, Piccinin AM, Mackinnon A, et al. (2006) Psychopathology in young people with intellectual disability. *JAMA* **296**, 1981–1989.

Emerson E (2003) Prevalence of psychiatric disorders in children and adolescents with and without intellectual disability. *J Intellect Disabil Res* **47**, 51–58.

Epel ES, Blackburn EH, Lin J, et al. (2004) Accelerated telomere shortening in response to life stress. *Proc Natl Acad Sci USA* **101**, 17212–17315.

Esbensen AJ, Benson BA (2006) A prospective analysis of life events, problem behaviours and depression in adults with intellectual disability. *J Intellect Disabil Res* **50**, 248–258.

Eskedal L, Hagemo P, Eskild A, Aamodt G, Selier KS, Thailow E (2004) A population-based study of extra-cardiac anomalies in children with congenital malformations. *Cardiol Young* **14**, 600–607.

Evenhuis HM (1996) Dutch consensus on diagnosis and treatment of hearing impairment in children and adults with intellectual disability. The Consensus Committee. *J Intellect Disabil Res* **40**, 451–456.

Farag TI, Teebi AS (1988) Possible evidence for genetic predisposition to nondisjunction in man. *J Med Genet* **25**, 136–137.

Fombonne E, Zakarian R, Bennett A, Meng L, McLean-Heywood D (2006) Pervasive developmental disorders in Montreal, Québec, Canada: prevalence and links with immunizations. *Pediatrics* **118**, e139–50.

Fong CT, Brodeur GM (1987) Down's syndrome and leukemia, epidemiology, genetics, cytogenetics and mechanisms of leukemogenesis. *Cancer Genet Cytogenet* **28**, 55–76.

Formigari R, di Donato RM, Gargiulo G, et al. (2004) Better surgical prognosis for patients with complete atrioventricular septal defect and Down's syndrome. *Ann Thorac Surg* **78**, 666–672.

Frid C, Drott P, Lundell B, Rasmussen F, Anneren G (1999) Mortality in Down's syndrome in relation to congenital malformations. *J Intellect Disabil Res* **43**, 234–241.

Frid C, Bjorkhem G, Jonzon A, Sunnegardh J, Anneren G, Lundell B (2004) Long-term survival in children with atrioventricular septal defect and common atrioventricular valvar orifice in Sweden. *Cardiol Young* **14**, 24–31.

Garrison MM, Jeffries H, Christakis DA (2005) Risk of death for children with Down syndrome and sepsis. *J Pediatr* **147**, 748–752.

Glasson EJ, Bittles AH (2008) The impact of ageing in people with intellectual and developmental disability. In: Bodzsár EB, Susanne C (eds) *Age Related Problems in Past and Present Populations*. Budapest: Plantin Publishing and Press, 27–43.

Glasson EJ, Hussain R (2008) Linked data. Opportunities and challenges in disability research. *J Intellect Dev Disabil* **33**, 285–291.

Glasson EJ, Sullivan SG, Hussain R, Petterson BA, Montgomery PD, Bittles AH (2002) The changing survival profile of people with Down's syndrome, implications for genetic counselling. *Clin Genet* **62**, 390–393.

Glasson EJ, Sullivan SG, Hussain R, Petterson BA, Montgomery PD, Bittles AH (2003) Comparative survival advantage of males with Down syndrome. *Am J Hum Biol* **15**, 192–195.

Goldacre MJ, Wotton CJ, Seagroatt V, Yeates D (2004) Cancers and immune related diseases associated with Down's syndrome, a record linkage study. *Arch Dis Child* **89**, 1014–1017.

Gustavson KH, Umb-Carlsson O, Sonnander K (2005) A follow-up study of mortality, health conditions and associated disabilities of people with intellectual disabilities in a Swedish county. *J Intellect Disabil Res* **49**, 905–914.

Hamamy HA, al-Hakkak ZS, al-Taha S (1990) Consanguinity and the genetic control of Down syndrome. *Clin Genet* **37**, 24–29.

Hartley SL, Maclean WE, Butler MG, Zarcone J, Thompson T (2005) Maladaptive behaviors and risk factors among the genetic subtypes of Prader–Willi syndrome. *AmJ Med Genet A* **136**, 140–145.

Hasle H, Haunstrup Clemmensen I, Mikkelsen M (2000) Risks of leukaemia and solid tumours in individuals with Down's syndrome. *Lancet* **355**, 165–169.

Hatton DD, Sideris J, Skinner M, et al. (2006) Autistic behavior in children with fragile X syndrome, prevalence, stability, and the impact of FMRP. *Am J Med Genet A* **140**, 1804–1813.

Hayes C, Johnson Z, Thornton L, et al. (1997) Ten-year survival of Down syndrome births. *Int J Epidemiol* **26**, 822–829.

Hill DA, Gridley G, Cnattingius S, et al. (2003) Mortality and cancer incidence among individuals with Down syndrome. *Arch Intern Med* **163**, 705–711.

Hogg J, Lucchino R, Wang K, Janicki M (2001) Healthy ageing – adults with intellectual disabilities, ageing and social policy. *J Appl Res Intellect Disabil* **14**, 229–255.

Holland AJ (2000) Ageing and learning disability. *Br J Psychiatry* **176**, 26–31.

Hou JW, Wang TR, Chuang SM (1998) An epidemiological and aetiological study of children with intellectual disability in Taiwan. *J Intellect Disabil Res* **42**, 137–143.

Huber B, Bocchicchio M, Hauser I, et al. (2009) Ambiguous results of an attempt to withdraw barbiturates in epilepsy patients with intellectual disability. *Seizure* **18(2)**, 109–118.

Hyman BT, West HL, Rebeck GW, Lai F, Mann DM (1995) Neuropathological changes in Down's syndrome hippocampal formation. Effect of age and apolipoprotein E genotype. *Arch Neurol* **52**, 373–378.

Jaffe JS, Timell AM, Elolia R, Thatcher SS (2005) Risk factors for low bone mineral density in individuals residing in a facility for the people with intellectual disability. *J Intellect Disabil Res* **49**, 457–462.

Janicki M, Dalton AJ (2000) Prevalence of dementia and impact on intellectual disability services. *Mental Retard* **38**, 276–288.

Janicki MP, Dalton AJ, Henderson CM, Davidson PW (1999) Mortality and morbidity among older adults with intellectual disability, health services considerations. *Disabil Rehab* **21**, 284–294.

Jobling A, Cuskelly M (2006) Young people with Down syndrome. A preliminary investigation of health knowledge and associated behaviours. *J Intellect Dev Disabil* **31**, 210–218.

Kandel I, Morad M, Vardi G, Merrick J (2005) Intellectual disability and parenthood *Scientif World J* **21**, 50–57.

Kerr AM, McCulloch D, Oliver K, et al. (2003) Medical needs of people with intellectual disability require regular reassessment, and the provision of client- and carer-held reports. *J Intellect Disabil Res* **47**, 134–145.

Keşer I, Canatan D, Güzeloglu-Kayisli O, Cosan R, Luleçi G (2001) Beta-thalassemia major associated with Down syndrome. *Annal Génétiq* **44**, 57–58.

Lai F, Roger S, Williams RS (1989) A prospective study of Alzheimer Disease in Down syndrome. *Arch Neurol* **46**, 849–853.

Leonard S, Bower C, Petterson B, Leonard H (2000) Survival of infants born with Down's syndrome, 1980–96. *Paediatr Perinat Epidemiol* **14**, 163–171.

Lo NS, Leung PM, Lau KC, Yeung CY (1989) Congenital cardiovascular malformations in Chinese children with Down's syndrome. *Chinese Med J* **102**, 382–386.

Lott IT, McGregor M, Engelman L, et al. (2004) Longitudinal prescribing patterns for psychoactive medications in community-based individuals with developmental disabilities, utilization of pharmacy records. *J Intellect Disabil Res* **48**, 563–571.

Mann DMA (1988) Alzheimer's disease and Down syndrome. *Histopathology* **13**, 125–137.

March of Dimes (2006) *Global Report on Birth Defects*. New York: March of Dimes.

Martens MA, Jones L, Reiss S (2006) Organ transplantation, organ donation and mental retardation. *Pediatr Transplant* **10**, 658–664.

Masuda M, Kado H, Tanoue Y, et al. (2005) Does Down syndrome affect the long-term results of complete atrioventricular septal defect when the defect is repaired during the first year of life? *Eur J Cardiothorac Surg* **27**, 405–409.

McCarron M, Gill M, McCallion P, Begley C (2005) Health co-morbidities in ageing persons with Down syndrome and Alzheimer's dementia. *J Intellect Disabil Res* **49**, 560–566.

McDermott S, Moran R, Platt T, Wood H, Isaac T, Dasari S (2005) Prevalence of epilepsy in adults with mental retardation and related disabilities in primary care. *Am J Mental Retard* **110**, 48–56.

Mehta PD, Capone G, Jewell A, Freedland RL (2007) Increased amyloid beta protein levels in children and adolescents with Down syndrome. *J Neurol Sci* **254**, 22–27.

Melville CA, Cooper SA, McGrother CW, Thorp CXF, Collacott R (2005) Obesity in adults with Down syndrome: a case-control study. *J Intellect Disabil Res* **49**, 125–133.

Melville CA, Cooper SA, Morrison J, et al. (2006) The outcomes of an intervention study to reduce the barriers experienced by people with intellectual disabilities accessing primary health care services. *J Intellect Disabil Res* **50**, 11–17.

Mencap (1998) *The NHS – Health For All? People with Learning Disabilities and Health Care*. London: Mencap.

Menéndez M (2005) Down syndrome, Alzheimer's disease and seizures. *Brain Dev* **27**, 246–252.

Menezes M, Puri P (2005) Long-term clinical outcome in patients with Hirschsprung's disease and associated Down's syndrome. *J Pediatr Surg* **40**, 810–812.

Metneki J, Czeizel AE (2005) Increasing total prevalence rate of cases with Down syndrome in Hungary. *Eur J Epidemiol* **20**, 525–535.

Meuwese-Jongejeugd A, van Splunder J, Vink M, et al. (2008) Combined sensory impairment (deaf-blindness) in five percent of adults with intellectual disabilities. *Am J Mental Retard* **113**, 254–262.

Milbrandt TA, Johnston CE (2005) Down syndrome and scoliosis, a review of a 50-year experience at one institution. *Spine* **30**, 2051–2055.

Morris J, Mutton D, Alberman E (2005) Corrections to maternal age-specific live birth prevalence of Down's syndrome. *J Med Screening* **12**, 202.

Myrelid A, Gustafsson J, Ollars B, Anneren G (2002) Growth charts for Down's syndrome from birth to 18 years of age. *Arch Dis Child* **87**, 97–103.

National Down Syndrome Society (2007) *Response to the American College of Obstetricians and Gynecologists' New Recommendations for Prenatal Testing*. www.ndss.org/index.php?option=com_content&view=article&id=153%3Aposition&limitstart=2.

National Health Service Cancer Screening Programme (2000) G*ood Practice in Breast and Cervical Screening for Women with Learning Disabilities*. Sheffield: National Health Service Cancer Screening Programmes, Publication no. 13.

Nicholson A, Alberman E (1992) Prediction of the number of Down's syndrome infants to be born in England and Wales up to the year 2000 and their likely survival rates. *J Intellect Disabil Res* **36**, 505–517.

Nirje B (1969a) A Scandinavian visitor looks at US institutions. In: Kugel RB, Wolfensberger W (eds) *Changing Patterns in Residential Services for the Mentally Retarded*. Washington, DC: President's Committee on Mental Retardation, pp. 51–57.

Nirje B (1969b) The normalization principle and its human management implications. In: Kugel RB, Wolfensberger W (eds) *Changing Patterns in Residential Services for the Mentally Retarded*. Washington, DC: President's Committee on Mental Retardation, pp. 179–195.

Nottestad JA, Linaker OM (1999) Psychiatric health needs and services before and after complete deinstitutionalization of people with intellectual disability. *J Intellect Disabil Res* **43**, 523–530.

Oberlander TF, Symons FJ (2006) *Pain in Children and Adults with developmental Disabilities*. Baltimore: Paul H. Brookes.

O'Leary P, Bower C, Murch A, Crowhurst J, Goldblatt J (1996) The impact of antenatal screening for Down syndrome in Western Australia, 1980–1994. *Aust NZ J Obstet Gynaecol* **36**, 385–388.

Olson LE, Richtsmeier JT, Leszl J, Reeves RH (2004) A chromosome 21 critical region does not cause specific Down syndrome phenotypes. *Science* **306**, 687–690.

Olson LE, Roper RJ, Sengstaken CL, et al. (2007) Trisomy for the Down syndrome "critical region" is necessary but not sufficient for brain phenotypes of trisomic mice. *Hum Mol Genet* **16**, 774–782.

Owens PL, Kerker BD, Zigler E, Horwitz SM (2006) Vision and oral health needs of individuals with intellectual disability. *Mental Retard Dev Disabil Res Rev* **12**, 28–40.

Patja K, Iivanainen M, Vesala H, Oksanen H, Ruoppila I (2000) Life expectancy of people with intellectual disability. A 35-year follow-up study. *J Intellect Disabil Res* **44**, 591–599.

Patja K, Eero P, Iivanainen M (2001) Cancer incidence among people with intellectual disability. *J Intellect Disabil Res* **45**, 300–307.

Penrose LS (1949) The incidence of Mongolism in the general population. *J Mental Sci* **95**, 685–688.

Piachaud J, Rohde J (1998) Screening for breast cancer is necessary in patients with learning disability. *BMJ* **316**, 1979–1980.

Polder JJ, Meerding WJ, Bonneux L, van der Maas PJ (2002) Healthcare costs of intellectual disability in the Netherlands, a cost-of-illness perspective. *J Intellect Disabil Res* **46**, 168–178.

Polednak AP (1977) Postmortem bacteriology and pneumonia in a mentally retarded population. *Am J Clin Pathol* **67**, 190–195.

Prasher V, Haque MS (2005) Misdiagnosis of thyroid disorders in Down syndrome, time to re-examine the myth. *Am J Mental Retard* **110**, 23–27.

Prasher VP, Chowdhury TA, Rowe BR, Bain SC (1997) ApoE genotype and Alzheimer's disease in adults with Down syndrome, meta-analysis. *Am J Mental Retard* **102**, 103–110.

Pueschel SM, Anneren G, Durlach R, Flores J, Sustrova M, Verma IC (1995) Guidelines for optimal care of persons with Down syndrome. *Acta Paediatr* **84**, 823–827.

Puri BK, Ho KW, Singh I (2001) Age of seizure onset in adults with Down's syndrome. *Int J Clin Pract* **55**, 442–444.

Rasmussen SA, Wong LY, Correa A, Gambrell D, Friedman JM (2006) Survival in infants with Down syndrome, Metropolitan Atlanta, 1979–1998. *J Pediatr* **148**, 806–812.

Record RG, Smith A (1955) Incidence, mortality, and sex distribution of mongoloid defectives. *Br J Prev Soc Med* **9**, 10–15.

Reller MD, Morris CD (1998) Is Down syndrome a risk factor for poor outcome after repair of congenital heart defects? *J Pediatr* **132**, 738–741.

Rimmer JH, Yamaki K (2006) Obesity and intellectual disability. *Mental Retard Dev Disabil Res Rev* **12**, 22–27.

Roberts DF, Roberts MJ, Johnston AW (1991) Genetic epidemiology of Down's syndrome in Shetland. *Hum Genet* **87**, 57–60.

Roeleveld N, Zielhuis GA, Gabreels F (1997) The prevalence of mental retardation, a critical review of recent literature. *Dev Med Child Neurol* **39**, 125–132.

Rogers NB, Hawkins BA, Eklund SJ (1998) The nature of leisure in the lives of older adults with intellectual disability. *J Intellect Disabil Res* **42**, 122–130.

Rosner BA, Hodapp RM, Fidler DJ, Sagun JN, Dykens EM (2004) Social competence in persons with Prader–Willi, Williams and Down's syndromes. *J Appl Res Intellect Disabil* **17**, 209–217.

Roussot MA, Lawrenson JB, Hewitson J, Smart R, de Decker HP (2006) Is cardiac surgery warranted in children with Down syndrome? A case-controlled review. *S Afr Med J* **96**, 924–930.

Satgé D, Sasco AJ (2002) Breast screening guidelines should be adapted in Down's syndrome. *BMJ* **324**, 1155.

Satgé D, Sommelet D, Geneix A, Nishi M, Malet P, Vekemans M (1998) A tumor profile in Down syndrome. *Am J Med Genet* **78**, 207–216.

Satgé D, Sasco AJ, Pujol H, Rethore MO (2001) Breast cancer in women with trisomy 21 (French). *Bull Acad Nat Med* **185**, 1239–1252.

Satgé D, Sasco AJ, Goldgar D, Vekemans M, Rethore MO (2004) A 23-year-old woman with Down syndrome, type 1 neurofibromatosis, and breast carcinoma. *Am J Med Genet* **125A**, 94–96.

Savulescu J (2001) Resources, Down's syndrome, and cardiac surgery. Do we really want "equality of access"? *BMJ* **322**, 875–876.

Schrager S (2006) Epidemiology of osteoporosis in women with cognitive impairment. *Mental Retard* **44**, 203–211.

Stoll C, Alembik Y, Dott B, Roth MP (1998) Study of Down syndrome in 238,942 consecutive births. *Annal Génét* **41**, 44–51.

Straetmans JM, van Schrojenstein Lantman-de Valk HM, Schellevis FG, Dinant GJ (2007) Health problems of people with intellectual disabilities: the impact for general practice. *Br J Gen Pract* **57**, 64–66.

Stromme P, Diseth TH (2000) Prevalence of psychiatric diagnoses in children with mental retardation, data from a population-based study. *Dev Med Child Neurol* **42**, 266–270.

Sullivan SG, Glasson EJ, Hussain R, et al. (2003) Breast cancer and the uptake of mammography screening services by women with intellectual disabilities. *Prev Med* **37**, 507–512.

Sullivan SG, Hussain R, Threlfall T, Bittles AH (2004) The incidence of cancer in people with intellectual disabilities. *Cancer Causes Control* **15**, 1021–1025.

Sullivan SG, Hussain R, Glasson EJ, Bittles AH (2007) The profile and incidence of cancer in Down syndrome. *J Intellect Disabil Res* **51**, 228–231.

Thomson AK, Glasson EJ, Bittles AH (2006) A long-term population-based clinical and morbidity review of Prader–Willi syndrome in Western Australia. *J Intellect Disabil Res* **50**, 69–78.

Toledo C, Alembik Y, Aguirre Jaime A, Stoll C (1999) Growth curves of children with Down syndrome. *Annal Génét* **42**, 81–90.

Tubman TR, Shields MD, Craig BG, Mulholland HC, Nevin NC (1991) Congenital heart disease in Down's syndrome, two year prospective early screening study. *BMJ* **302**, 1425–1427.

Tuffrey-Wijne I (2003) The palliative care needs of people with intellectual disabilities, a literature review. *Palliat Med* **17**, 55–62.

US Public Health Service (2001) *Closing the Gap. A National Blueprint for Improving the Health of Individuals with Mental Retardation*. Report of the Surgeon General's Conference on Health Disparities and Mental Retardation. Washington, DC.

Van Allen MI, Fung J, Jurenka SB (1999) Health care concerns and guidelines for adults with Down syndrome. *Am J Med Genet* **89**, 100–110.

Van den Akker M, Maaskant MA, van der Meijden RJ (2006) Cardiac diseases in people with intellectual disability. *J Intellect Disabil Res* **50**, 515–522.

Van Splunder J, Stilma JS, Bernsen RM, Evenhuis HM (2006) Prevalence of visual impairment in adults with intellectual disabilities in The Netherlands, cross-sectional study. *Eye* **20**, 1004–1010.

Venugopalan P, Agarwal AK (2003) Spectrum of congenital heart defects associated with Down Syndrome in high consanguineous Omani population. *Indian Pediatr* **40**, 398–403.

Vida VL, Barnoya J, Larrazabal LA, Gaitan G, de Maria Garcia F, Castaneda AR (2005) Congenital cardiac disease in children with Down's syndrome in Guatemala. *Cardiolog Young* **15**, 286–290.

Visser FE, Aldenkamp AP, van Huffelen AC, Kuilman M, Overweg J, van Wijk J (1997) Prospective study of the prevalence of Alzheimer-type dementia in institutionalized individuals with Down syndrome. *Am J Mental Retard* **101**, 400–412.

Wallace RA, Webb PM, Schluter PJ (2002) Environmental, medical, behavioural and disability factors associated with *Helicobacter pylori* infection in adults with intellectual disability. *J Intellect Disabil Res* **46**, 51–60.

Wellesley D, Hockey A, Stanley F (1991) The aetiology of intellectual disability in Western Australia, a community-based study. *Dev Med Child Neurol* **33**, 963–973.

Wells GL, Barker SE, Finley SC, Colvin EV, Finley WH (1994) Congenital heart disease in infants with Down's syndrome. *South Med J* **87**, 724–727.

World Health Organization (2000) *Ageing and Intellectual Disabilities – Improving Longevity and Promoting Healthy Ageing, Summative Report*. Geneva: World Health Organization.

World Health Organization (2001) *The World Health Report 2001*. Geneva: World Health Organization.

Zigman W, Schupf N, Haveman M, Silverman W (1997) The epidemiology of Alzheimer disease in intellectual disability. Results and recommendations from an international conference. *J Intellect Disabil Res* **41**, 76–80.

10
COMORBIDITY: CLASSIFICATION ARTEFACT AND CLINICAL REALITY

Rutger Jan van der Gaag

Comorbidity is a term commonly used in (developmental psycho-) pathology but it has only come into fashion recently (Caron & Rutter 1991). Of the some 900 articles with the term as keyword found in PubMed, over 700 were published in the last 10 years. In this chapter, the question will be addressed whether this represents a changing reality in psychopathology or whether this immense increase merely reflects an artefact caused by the current classification systems and the way in which in Western society they are used by researchers but also clinicians, medical insurance companies and policy makers.

Nevertheless it will become clear that clinicians are often confronted with cases that require attention to interfering processes (called comorbid conditions) that make it difficult to adhere to the mainstream approach of the first condition considered. Thus it will be concluded that despite the theoretical discussion on the usefulness of the concept of comorbidity, it is a clinical reality that requires attention in practice and in training.

Comorbidity as a question of definition
The term 'comorbidity' is used for different relationships between 'morbid' conditions. These conditions may be circumscribed illnesses, developmental or psychiatric disorders. In general, five possibilities exist. The term 'comorbidity' may be used:

- to signal the co-occurrence of two distinct conditions, e.g. a somatic condition (pneumonia) requiring treatment in a patient hospitalised for a psychosis. In this case, comorbidity reflects a coincidence
- to focus attention on two different aspects of one condition that might require attention in their own right: anxiety and sleep problems in a depression
- to draw attention to the frequent co-occurrence of two conditions, suggesting that there could be a relation between them, without speculating on the nature of that relationship, e.g. attention-deficit–hyperactivity disorder (ADHD) is far more common in patients with Tourette disorder. The questions here are: (1) is there a genetic connection between the two conditions or (2) do the two conditions overlap on the basis of an impulsivity issue common to both?
- to suggest a supposed causal effect: if one has condition A, one is more likely to also or subsequently develop condition B. For example, a child with severe ADHD could start experimenting with drugs in adolescence, making it likely that he would develop a comorbid substance abuse condition along with the ADHD

- to point to time development track interaction: it is a well-established fact that children with ADHD may develop display oppositional defiant behaviour that later may turn into antisocial conduct disorders.
- The four last examples are from psychiatry and for good reasons: the rise of interest in and articles on comorbidity seem to coincide with a radical change in classification systems (ICD and DSM) in the early 1980s, thus possibly reflecting an artefact rather than a real change. In psychopathology diagnosis and classification are not synonymous. This needs some explanation if we want to understand the apparent surge of comorbidity properly.

On classification and diagnosis

Diagnosis is a clinical term and refers to the comprehensive summary of the information gathered during the examination that will inform the 'patient' and their family about the nature of the condition, treatment possibilities and what may be expected in terms of recovery and outcome. The clinician is confident about statements made on the nature, treatment possibilities and prognosis not because of their knowledge of this particular case but because of the connection they make between this case and the scientific knowledge and evidence available on comparable cases: the 'class' of cases. This knowledge is available through international classification systems.

Classifying is well embedded in human nature and appears naturally during the second year of life when infants start gathering objects and becoming interested in similarities and differences. In science classification is of uttermost importance, Linnaeus started classifying the plants for scientific purposes. Medicine followed in the 19th century. Yet in the beginning medicine was less fortunate than biology because in most cases, the relation between the complaints, symptoms and signs was far from obvious. The positivists proposed meticulous descriptions in search of meaningful associations between different signs, thus starting to describe syndromes as associations of signs that did not occur only by chance. But these pertinent clinical descriptions did not differentiate between diseases that superficially were similar but had different causes. A well-known example is tuberculosis and sarcoidosis. Both diseases present with casifying tubercles that may be apparent in different organs but a differentiation was not possible on a purely clinical basis. Blood parameters allowing differentiation between an infection and an autoimmunological condition were not available. So a great advance was made when Louis Pasteur discovered the tubercle bacillus that causes tuberculosis and is not present in sarcoidosis, as described by Besnier and Boek. So the advance that was meaningful in this case, as in so many in medicine, was the identification of the cause or at least of the main causal factor.

But in developmental psychopathology things are less clear-cut as none of the conditions described in the psychopathology sections of the classification systems have only one single cause. On the contrary – the behavioural expression of a condition results from intricate transactional processes at many different levels. These transactional processes with ongoing interactions over time thus shape the development of the individual.

In fact, the interactions between gene and environment start from the first meiosis. The very early circumstances within the womb will influence embryogenesis in a beneficial or

Genetic (pre)disposition

⇑⇓   ⇔ *Womb-environment*

Epigenetic phenomena

⇑⇓   ⇔ *(Womb) environment*

Functional pathways - neurotransmitters

⇑⇓   ⇔ *Environment*

Neurocognitive profile
Information-processing style / capacities

⇑⇓   ⇔ *Environment*

Invisible but testable

Visible phenotype and interactions
Behavioural phenotype

⇑⇓

Social context - environment

Figure 10.1 Transactional processes in development.

detrimental fashion. For developmental psychopathology, the first 16 weeks of gestation are very important. In that period, all the major circuits in the nervous system will be wired up, prepared to respond to external stimulation when that becomes available. The visual system will develop if stimulated by the excitation of the optical fibres when exposed to light. Similarly, the regions of the brain prepared for the processing of language and speech will respond to the stimulation of being spoken to. But the response of the infant has a major impact on the amount of stimulation to which it is exposed: the happy child who laughs cheerfully in response to babbling adults around the sixth week of life will encourage the adults to interact with him. Conversely, the child who seems bored when spoken to will 'discourage' the adult who in return will become less and less talkative.

Responsiveness and temperament are regulated by central mechanisms in the thalamus and determine the number of synapses that are joined in the information-processing activities in the brain. So from a developmental point of view, the genes in interaction with the environment determine the structural configuration of the brain. In turn, the structure will develop in interaction with the environment, thus configuring the 'neurotransmitter' make-up of the individual's brain. Likewise, stress management circuits, including hormonal feedback loops such as the hypothalamus-pituary-adrenocortical axis, will be influenced by external circumstances. For example, early trauma may have lasting effects but the expression of that imbalance may be very different. In some, it will enhance the likelihood of substance abuse in adolescence; in others, it may express itself in recurring depressive episodes in adulthood.

Between these neurophysiological endophenotypes and the behavioural pathology is another layer that must be taken into account: the neurocognitive make-up. Along with intelligence, other cognitive organising principles will contribute to the adaptive potential of an individual: the executive functions that determine one's capacity for flexible adaptation, planning and organising activities, the sense of central coherence that enables an individual to understand the complex surrounding world: both globally and in detail when appropriate. These functions will be mediated by intelligence but also by underlying important functions such as attention (selection, inhibition, attention span, distractability), impulsivity and the potential for postponing reward when circumstances thus dictate.

When one considers the intricate complexity of these interactions within the individual, on one hand, and between the individual and the environment, one is astonished by the fact that most individuals are so extremely resilient and capable of adapting to continuously changing circumstances. When the development follows a deviant pathway it may be obvious that the behavioural expression of dysfunction will be very different from one individual to another. For instance, under persisting stress one individual will become anxious, perhaps shifting to obsessions or a depressed mood, whilst another may react in a completely different manner, becoming oppositional and aggressive. Conversely, attentional problems may lead to different clinical pictures ranging from ADHD and schizophrenia to depression. This means that from a clinical point of view, one has to be cautious: different behavioural manifestations may stem from one underlying mechanism – anxiety, aggression and mood are mediated by the same neurotransmitter, serotonin. Different behaviours described as comorbidity at clinical level may be in fact very closely linked at a neurophysiological level.

So where diagnosing is concerned, the clinician will try and integrate the disturbances, strengths and weaknesses at different levels into a diagnostic formulation that will explain why these symptoms occur in this individual given their potential and developmental profile in transaction with their environment from a broad perspective (biological, psychological and socio-economical).

But when it comes to classifying this diagnosis, the current classification systems laid out in the *Diagnostic and Statistical Manual of Mental Disorders* (DSM, currently 4th revised edition, 2004) and the *International Classification of Diseases* (ICD, currently 10th edition, 1994) offer far fewer possibilities. Beginning with DSM-III back in 1981, the psychiatric classifications were only based on a-theoretical facts that could be observed or noted in a reliable fashion, independently from professional or theoretical (psychodynamic, behaviouristic or neurobiological) perspectives. Thus the categories were reduced to observable clinical classes. The behavioural criteria were initially based on expert consensus as were the cut-off points as to how many positive criteria were required to 'qualify' for the condition. In the latest versions (DSM-IV (Diagnostic and Statistical Manual of Mental Disorders, 4th edition) and ICD-10 (International Statistical Classification of Diseases and Related Disorders, 10 revision)), so-called field trials (e.g. Barkley 2003, Lahey et al. 1994) were conducted, giving more empirically based cut-off scores reflecting an optimum for sensitivity and specificity. Yet the criteria were still a matter of expert consensus. Consensus is not always the best way of searching for empirical truth. How futile the results of such discussions sometimes may be is illustrated by the following joke and on the case of Asperger. What is a camel? The answer is 'a horse, defined by a committee!'. The case of Asperger syndrome within DSM-IV is even more cynical. One may wonder why a proper name should be used to define a syndrome but given that, the committee could have taken a close look at the original account by the author himself or at carefully distilled criteria such as those suggested by Szatmari (1992) and Gillberg (1998). But the committee decided to take a shortcut and defined Asperger syndrome according to DSM-IV as autistic disorder without any positive criteria on the dimension 'communication'. The result is tragi-comic: Miller & Ozonoff (1997) applied the DSM-IV rules to the original case descriptions by Asperger and realised that none of them, according to the classification rules, qualified for the condition but had to be classified as autistic disorder because, despite their verbal abilities, the patients' reciprocal communicative skills were so poor that they had to be acknowledged at some point along the criteria for communication within the DSM criteria for pervasive developmental disorders.

Comorbidity as clinical reality

If it is true that part of the comorbidity question reflects a classification artefact, the other side of the coin is that clinical cases are seldom clear-cut. Taking autism as an example, comorbidity is more rule than exception: more than 80% of all individuals classified with an autistic disorder also meet the criteria for an anxiety disorder, more than 60% have aggressive outbursts at some time, 50% present with hyperactivity. These could be classified on axis one representing a clinical condition. On axis two, in many cases an intellectual disability could be classified. However, clinically, hyper- or hyposensitivities to noise, light, pain or temperature cannot be classified, not because they do not exist but because they are not acknowledged as a distinct disorder. Yet in clinical practice these sensitivities are encountered very often as a major problem, a clinical challenge that needs a solution as this can be a tremendous burden for the individual with autism.

Looking back at the questions of multiple levels of (dys)functioning, both the comorbidities and the non-classifiable sensitivities can be conceived of as distinct but it is more likely that they are manifestations of the dysfunctioning in autism at different levels. In autism, anxiety is not a distinct condition but a symptom of distress. On can hypothesise that the anxieties stem from the cognitive information-processing deficits. The individual cannot predict situations and gets anxious. The aggressive outburst could be a reaction to the anxiety. The hyper- and hyposensitivities could reflect disorders in the arousal regulation at one level higher. Thus defined, these conditions would not be comorbid in the sense that they need attention in their own right as distinct disorders, but they are manifestations of a high level of stress and require that clinicians pay attention to the basic programme they are offering to help the individual to cope with the problems stemming from the autism. In that case, the comorbid anxiety and aggression are signals that should urge those who provide treatment and guidance to take a close look at their interventions and the daily schedules to ensure that these are clear and consistent and provide enough security for the individual involved.

But in other cases a comorbid classification can be subject to treatment in its own right. For example, if a youngster admitted with substance use disorder (SUD), after detoxification appears to meet the criteria for ADHD, which according to the history taken from the parents was present from toddlerhood on, this underlying disorder will need to be treated according to the protocols with stimulant medication and psychoeducation. By doing so, the chance of relapsing into SUD will drop dramatically (Wilens 2007).

These two examples underscore the necessity for clinicians to take assessment seriously and to think in terms of diagnosis – understanding why different symptoms co-occur – rather than classification.

Future directions

Diagnosing remains the core activity of clinicians. Classification, on the other hand, is essential for three good reasons.

- *Communication* – referring to a classification helps clinicians communicate more quickly and with precision.
- *Control* – the discipline of classifying according to the rules but also reclassifying after a period of intervention helps to monitor for progress, deterioration or shifting into other conditions. Thus classification has an important monitoring function.
- *Comprehension* – classification is of the utmost importance for scientific progress. Studies will be comparable if the inclusion criteria for a certain condition are comparable: in other words, if research groups apply the same classification criteria as inclusion and exclusion criteria for study groups and eventual contrast groups.

Unequal access to services is a threat to classification systems. Many insurance companies, special services and schools nowadays require classifications to qualify for their services or admittance into schools. On one hand, one can understand policy makers wanting to use 'objective criteria' to allocate a fair share of provisions. But on the other hand, this is misuse of a system that has often been tailored merely for clinical and scientific use.

So how should we approach the future?

FOR CLASSIFICATION SYSTEMS

ICD-10 has a clinical and a research version. For the future this seems to become an even more important issue to prevent misuse of scientific systems by policy makers. Another issue in developmental psychopathology is that of the multiaxial system. Now distinctions are made between (1) clinical conditions, (2) intelligence and personality, (3) somatic conditions, (4) psychosocial stress and (5) a global assessment of functioning. Given the scientific progress pointing at different interacting levels in developmental psychopathology, one might consider the possibility of including 'endophenotypes' at different levels (e.g. impulsivity, weak inhibition, detailed perception) to encourage studies that could shed light on differences and similarities in clinical manifestations of the same underlying neuropsychological deviance. Interestingly, the need for impairment measures and a reappraisal of comorbidity is open to discussion in the interactive tailoring of DSM-V: http://www.dsm5.org/.

FOR CLINICAL PRACTICE

Scientific progress based on sound classification helps clincians to understand the nature and course of disorders that they encounter in clinical practice. Clear-cut cases are rare and generally speaking, clinicians will be confronted with mixed pictures – in other words, with individuals who display many comorbid conditions. The classification systems will help to define these different clinical features but critical clinical appraisal is still vital in weighing the importance of each condition and in determining the hierarchy of symptoms and syndromes in order to tailor a comprehensive treatment programme adjusted to the needs of the individual in the context of family environment and broader psychosocial setting.

REFERENCES

Barkley RA (2003) Issues in the diagnosis of attention-deficit/hyperactivity disorder in children. *Brain Dev* **25**(2), 77–83.

Caron C, Rutter M (1991) Comorbidity in child psychopathology: concepts, issues and research strategies. *J Child Psychol Psychiatr* **32**(7), 1063–1080.

Gillberg C (1998) Asperger syndrome and high-functioning autism. *Br J Psychiatr* **172**, 200–209.

Lahey BB, Applegate B, McBurnett K, et al. (1994) DSM-IV field trials for attention deficit hyperactivity disorder in children and adolescents. *Am J Psychiatr* **151**(11), 1673–1685.

Miller JN, Ozonoff S (1997) Did Asperger's cases have Asperger disorder? A research note. *J Child Psychol Psychiatr* **38**(2), 247–251.

Szatmari P (1992) The validity of autistic spectrum disorders: a literature review. *J Autism Dev Disord* **22**(4), 583–600.

Wilens TE (2007) The nature of the relationship between attention-deficit/hyperactivity disorder and substance use. *J Clin Psychiatr* **11**(Suppl), 4–8.

INDEX

Note: page numbers in *italics* refer to figures and tables

149